RAND

Variations in the Use of Cesarean Sections:

Literature Synthesis

Joanna Zorn Heilbrunn, Rolla Edward Park

Prepared for the
Agency for Health Care Policy and Research

PREFACE

This research is part of the Management and Outcomes of Childbirth Patient Outcomes Research Team (PORT), which is supported by the Agency for Health Care Policy and Research. This report summarizes the literature on variations in the use of cesarean section for childbirth, including variations over time, geographic variations, and clinical and nonclinical correlates of variations and should be of interest to those researching childbirth and C-sections. The larger project includes literature syntheses on other topics such as outcomes of C-section versus vaginal birth, and costs of delivery. It will also include analyses of secondary data to estimate the probability of getting a C-section, and also to estimate outcomes (morbidity, mortality, length of stay, readmissions) as a function of similar variables together with method of delivery. In addition, we will use decision analysis to formulate guidelines for the appropriate use of C-section, and test interventions that may result in more-appropriate use.

This report was largely completed in August 1993; final publication has been delayed. Since August 1993, several important studies of variations in cesarean section rates have appeared. We have not attempted to include the recent studies in our review, but we have listed the ones that we are aware of following the references.

CONTENTS

TABLES

ACKNOWLEDGMENTS

We are grateful to Marjorie Pearson, who worked with RAND library staff to conduct the computerized literature searches. We also appreciate helpful reviews and comments on the draft report by Olivia A. Crookes, Cedars-Sinai Medical Center, and Robert M. Bell, RAND.

1. INTRODUCTION

FRAMEWORK FOR THIS LITERATURE SYNTHESIS

This report summarizes the literature on variations in the use of cesarean section for childbirth, including variations over time, geographic variations, and clinical and nonclinical correlates of variations. We think of variations in C-section rates in a multivariate regression framework. In this framework, the probability that a mother delivering a baby in a hospital will have a C-section is a function of

- mother's characteristics, such as:
  - -- current clinical data (diagnoses, health status, etc.)
  - -- historical clinical data (age, previous birth history, etc.)
  - -- demographic data (race, education, etc.)
  - -- economic data (income, insurance, etc.)

- physician's characteristics, such as
  - -- demographic data (age, sex, race, etc.)
  - -- professional data (training, certification, experience, etc.)
  - -- practice (solo, group, HMO, etc.)
  - -- practice style (propensity to perform elective cesareans)

- hospital's characteristics, such as
  - -- ownership (for profit, not for profit, public, etc.)
  - -- teaching status
  - -- size (number of beds, etc.)
  - -- location (urban, rural, etc.)
  - -- practice style (propensity to perform elective cesareans)

- temporal and geographic factors not otherwise measured
  - -- year
  - -- state

-- country

-- etc.

If we have enough individual-level data on the above variables from enough different settings, we can estimate a series of logistic regressions that would encapsulate most of what one might want to know about variations. No one has analyzed such a complete data set, but the literature may be thought of as a set of partial regressions, each focusing on only one or a few of the relationships listed. For example, simple time series that describe the increase in C-section rates involve only years as independent variables. Some small-area variations studies involve only cities or zip codes. Many studies in the literature report C-section rates as functions of year and diagnosis. Other studies examine the effect of hospital characteristics on C-section rates after controlling for some patient characteristics.

OBJECTIVES OF THE LITERATURE SYNTHESIS

This synthesis of the literature on variations in C-section rates is part of a much larger project. The larger project includes literature syntheses on other topics, such as outcomes of C-section versus vaginal birth, and costs of delivery. It will also include analyses of secondary data to estimate the probability of getting a C-section in regressions like those outlined above, and also to estimate outcomes (morbidity, mortality, length of stay, readmissions) as a function of similar variables together with method of delivery. In addition, we will use decision analysis to formulate guidelines for the appropriate use of C-section and test interventions that may result in more-appropriate use.

The variations literature synthesis is meant to support the larger project in the following specific ways:

1. To synthesize what is known about the effect of any of the above factors on probability of C-section; to serve as a description of "what is" for comparison with the "what ought to be" from the decision analysis.

2. To guide the secondary data analysis by gathering information on factors that are known to affect C-section rates importantly, and on appropriate ways to model those factors.
3. To identify gaps in what is known about "what is" that we may be able to fill with our secondary data analysis.

THE COMPUTER SEARCH

We started our literature synthesis by conducting three searches of computer databases. The searches were intended to find articles that contained information on rates of use of C-sections and other obstetrical interventions.

Search 1: Search the MEDLINE databases (covering articles published during 1966 through June 1991) for articles whose descriptive words, titles, or abstracts, contain words that match:
(CESAREAN SECTION or
VAGINAL BIRTH AFTER CESAREAN or
VBAC)

and

(RATES or
VARIATION or
UTILIZATION or
TRENDS or
STATISTICAL AND NUMERICAL DATA).

Search 2: Search the MEDLINE databases (covering articles published during 1966 through June 1991) for articles whose descriptive words and titles (but not abstracts), contain words that match:

(DELIVERY or
EPISIOTOMY or
EXTRACTION, OBSTETRICAL or
VACUUM EXTRACTION, OBSTETRICAL or

HOME CHILDBIRTH or
LABOR, INDUCED or
NATURAL CHILDBIRTH or
VAGINAL BIRTH AFTER CESAREAN or
VERSION, FETAL or
LABOR or
LABOR ONSET or
LABOR STAGE, FIRST or
LABOR STAGE, SECOND or
LABOR STAGE, THIRD or
TRIAL OF LABOR or
UTERINE CONTRACTION or
OBSTETRICAL FORCEPS)
and
(RATES or
VARIATION or
UTILIZATION or
TRENDS or
STATISTICAL AND NUMERICAL DATA).

Search 3: Search the Health Planning and Administration database (covering articles published during 1975 through June 1991) for articles whose descriptive words, titles, or abstracts, contain words that match:

(CESAREAN SECTION or
VAGINAL BIRTH AFTER CESAREAN or
VBAC)
or
(DELIVERY or
EPISIOTOMY or
EXTRACTION, OBSTETRICAL or
VACUUM EXTRACTION, OBSTETRICAL or
HOME CHILDBIRTH or
LABOR, INDUCED or
NATURAL CHILDBIRTH)

and
(RATES or
VARIATION or
UTILIZATION or
TRENDS or
STATISTICAL AND NUMERICAL DATA).

SELECTING ARTICLES OF POSSIBLE INTEREST

The computer searches produced lists of thousands of titles. We read through the lists and marked those that appeared to be relevant to the variations literature synthesis. We marked citations that seemed from the title as though they might have information on geographic or temporal variations in C-section rates, or clinical or nonclinical determinates or correlates of C-section rates. The computer search turned up almost nothing on variations in other obstetrical interventions; we excluded any such articles because there were not enough to support any kind of systematic review.

We also excluded editorials, letters, opinion pieces, and single-hospital studies, insofar as it was possible to identify them from the computer listings. Initially we also excluded non-U.S. and non-Canada studies with no North American comparison.

Search 1 produced a list of 1340 titles; we marked 106 of them as being of possible interest and obtained copies of those 106.

Search 2 produced a list of 1660 titles; we marked 91 of them as being of possible interest. Of the 91, 69 duplicated titles already chosen for copying from the list for search 1. We obtained copies of the unduplicated 22.

Search 3 produced a list of 83 titles; we marked only 2 of them as being of possible interest. One of the 2 duplicated an article already chosen from the list for search 1; we obtained a copy of the other one.

After writing the first draft of this report, we decided to include a section on international cesarean rates. We looked through the searches a second time, marking titles that named other countries or regions. We selected and copied an additional set of 40 articles from the searches.

We obtained a few additional articles in two other ways. First, we scanned the bibliographies and reference lists in the copied articles, looking for articles of apparent interest that we had not already copied. We found 21 additional articles in this way. Second, other literature review teams referred us to a few articles that they thought might be relevant to our variations review. We obtained 12 articles from the other teams.

It was not always possible to spot the intended exclusion criteria (single-hospital study, etc.) from the title alone; we excluded citations that were copied as soon as we identified them based on the article itself. A total of 121 articles were dropped after copying because upon inspection they were found to meet our exclusion criteria, or else not to include any new information relevant to variations in C-section rates. The remaining 81 articles used in this literature synthesis are cited in the references section of this report.

2. TEMPORAL AND GEOGRAPHICAL VARIATIONS IN TOTAL CESAREAN RATES

INTERNATIONAL VARIATIONS

Although rates of cesarean delivery by country seem to have risen universally during the 1970s and early 1980s, there is great disparity in national rates; the United States has been among the highest for years. In one study of 19 countries, the U.S. rate was the highest from 1973 through 1983, with Canada close behind (Notzon, Placek, and Taffel, 1987). A 21-country study shows the 1985 U.S. rate of 23 percent to be lower than only the Brazilian 32 percent and Puerto Rican 29 percent rates. Switzerland, New Zealand, England and Wales, the Netherlands, Hungary, Japan, and Czechoslovakia all had rates less than one-half of the U.S. rate in that year. Of these countries, only Hungary and Czechoslovakia had higher perinatal mortality rates (Notzon, 1990). Although medical indications may differ across populations, these figures suggest that the United States has much room to lower its C-section rate without compromising quality of care.

Table 1 shows cesarean rates for 29 countries. Each line in the table represents data from one source. A source here refers to any number of publications based on the same data and written by the same author(s), or even by different authors as long as they arrived at the same results. Citations are listed by reference code in the bibliography. The letter is the first letter of the first author's last name, and the number indicates the alphabetical rank of the article among all those beginning with the same initial. Blanks indicate that no data were presented by the source for the given year. Note that not every rate covers the entire country. Some are based on a state or region; a few report only one, albeit major, hospital.

Rates for two or more years are presented for only 23 of these countries or regions, so we know little about cesarean use in most of the world. There are notable gaps in our table, even regarding the industrialized world. We have French and Japanese rates for only four years, and no data at all for Germany, for example. It is likely that

Table 1

International Cesarean Section Rates, by Year

Country	Ref	1970	1971	1972	1973	1974	1975	1976	1977	1978	1979	1980	1981	1982	1983	1984	1985	1986	1987	1988	1989	1990
Australia	N4	4.2	4.1	4.6	5.1	7.3	8.2	8.7	9.9	11.7	13.0	13.2	14.0									
**	N3																16					
	R3																	16.9				
Western Australia	R3																	15.1				
Western Australia	R1											11.2	11.8	12.5	13.3	13.9	15.1	15.6	16.9			
New South Wales	R3																	16.0				
Victoria	R3																	16.5				
South Australia	R3																	18.2				
South Australia	J1												16.9	17.4	18.7	17.7	17.9	18.9				
Queensland	R3																	18.4				
Northern Territory	R3																	19.8				
Australian Capital Territory	R3																	26.3				
Austria	N4												6.5	7.0	7.5							
Bavaria	N4										11.3	11.2	11.7	12.2	13.2							
**	N3																15					
Belgium	N4												7.4	8.0	8.1							
	B2										7.2											
Brazil **	N3												[		32			]				
Urban hospitals in Paraiba	R3								19.0	20.9	24.7	26.8	28.5									
State of Rio Grande do Norte	R3											17.6										
State of Pernambuco	R3											16.8										
Canada	N4,W1	5.7	6.4	7.2	8.0	9.0	9.6	10.8	12.1	13.9	15.1	15.9										
*	L2	6.0	6.4	7.2	8.0	9.0	9.6	10.8	12.1	13.9	14.7	15.2	15.8									
**	N3															[19	]					
Colombia, urban hospitals **	L3								7.1													
Czechoslovakia	N4	2.3	2.3	2.4	2.5	2.6	2.8	3.1	3.4	3.7	4.0	4.4	4.7	5.2	6.0							
	N3																7					
	L2												4.0									
	B2										4.0											
Denmark	N4	5.7		5.9		7.2	7.5	8.0	8.8		9.0		11.7	11.7	12.8							
	N3																13					
	L2										10.7											
	B2										10.3											

Table 1--continued

Country	Ref	1970	1971	1972	1973	1974	1975	1976	1977	1978	1979	1980	1981	1982	1983	1984	1985	1986	1987	1988	1989	1990
England & Wales	N4	5.0	5.2	5.3	5.3	5.6	6.0	6.5	7.4	7.5	8.5	9.0	9.3	10.1	10.1							
	L2	4.3	4.6	4.9	5.0	5.3	5.7	6.3	7.1	7.3	8.2	8.8	9.1									
	N3																10					
Finland	N4	6.0	6.9	7.2	7.9	8.1	8.2	8.8	10.0	10.9	11.9											
	L2										11.9											
	B2										11.9											
France	N4			6.1				8.5					10.9									
	L2												10.7									
**	B2										8.0											
Greece	N3																13					
Hungary	N4	6.2	6.7	6.9	7.0	6.7	6.5	6.6	6.9	7.4	7.6	8.0	8.6	9.2	9.5							
	N3																10					
•	B2									8.0												
India, Calcutta, 1 hospital	D1	2.5 (1970-71)										5.4 (1980-81)										
India, Manipur State	S5			3.0	3.8	2.4	3.2	2.7	3.7	5.5												
Israel †	M8														9.6							
Italy	N3													13								
Italy, Latium region	B3																22.5					
Japan	N4						6.4	6.5	6.8				8.0									
	N3																7					
Netherlands																						
all deliveries	N4	2.1	2.1	2.2	2.5	2.6	2.7	2.9	3.5	3.8	4.3	4.7	4.9	5.3								
hospitals only	N4	5.3	5.1	5.3	5.6	5.9	5.9	5.9	7.0	7.4	8.2	8.9	9.4	10.5	11.4							
Netherlands	L2	2.0	2.1	2.3	2.5	2.7	2.8	2.9	3.5	3.9	3.9	4.3	4.7									
	B2									3.6												
	N3																10					
New Zealand	N4	3.9		3.9	5.2	5.0		5.2					9.7	9.8								
	L1														9.6							
	N3																10					
Norway	N4	2.2	2.4	2.5	3.0	3.6	4.1	5.0	6.4	7.3	8.0	8.3	8.7	9.0	9.4							
††	B4	2.4			4.0			6.2			8.3			9.7								
	L2										8.3											
	B2										8.0											
	N3																12					
Poland •	B2									5.0												

Table 1--continued

Country	Ref	1970	1971	1972	1973	1974	1975	1976	1977	1978	1979	1980	1981	1982	1983	1984	1985	1986	1987	1988	1989	1990
Portugal	N4	6.1	7.2	8.3	7.9	8.7	8.9	8.4	9.1	9.1	10.3	9.5	9.4	9.8	12.9							
••	N3																		13			
Puerto Rico	N3														[	29	]					
Rumania •	B2									4.6												
Saudi Arabia, Riyadh Δ	C2										3.9	5.4	6.0	5.4	7.5	9.9						
Scotland ΔΔ	N4	5.9	6.6	7.2	7.5	8.2	8.5	9.5	10.1	10.8	11.4	11.7	12.0	12.8								
	L2										10.7											
§	B2									10.7												
	N3																14					
Spain ••	N3																12					
Sweden	N4				5.5	6.8	7.8	9.6	10.9	11.6	11.7	12.1	12.4									
	M6				5.5	6.8	7.8	9.6	10.9	11.3	11.9											
	L2										12.0											
	B2										11.7											
	N3																12					
Switzerland ••	N3														[	11		]				
US	N4,P2,P3,T1,T2,V2	5.5	5.8	7.0	8.0	9.2	10.4	12.1	13.7	15.2	16.4	16.5	17.9	18.5	20.3	21.1	22.7	24.1	24.4	24.7	23.8	23.5
	S2	5.7				9.2				14.7						21.2						
	S3										14.1					19.0						
	N3																23					
Zaire, Kasongo district	S2																					
Urban women 1976-1984	S2							[				1.1				]						
Rural women 1976-1984	S2							[				0.3				]						
Zimbabwe, Gweru Hospital §§	D4											(1982-1984)		16.8		8.0 (1984-1986)						

* 1979-1981 adjustments for Quebec are absent causing a probable underestimation of about 1.5%.

** Based on samples.

• Based on either 1977, 1978 or 1979 data.

•• Based on incomplete coverage.

† Rate is based on 11/1/83-1/31/84.

†† Based on three-year averages beginning with the year indicated.

Δ Data are for the Maternity and Children's Hospital serving 70% of the hospital births in Riyadh.

ΔΔ 1970-1974 rates are based on incomplete coverage and are probably overestimated.

§ Rate is for single births only.

§§ A successful intervention to lower c-section rates was carried out in this provincial hospital.

many countries, particularly less-developed ones, do not keep statistics on method of birth. It is also likely that English-language medical journals do not report all the information that is collected. Either way, it is clear that care providers in this country do not have easy access to information concerning birthing practices elsewhere.

In 1970, the U.S. rate of 5.5 percent was about average compared with that of other nations. Of the 13 countries for which we have data, six had rates slightly higher than that of the United States; they were Hungary, Portugal, Finland, Canada, Scotland, and Denmark, in roughly that order. Norway, the Netherlands, and the hospital in Calcutta, India, had the lowest rates. Cesarean sections became more common over time in all but one country--Zimbabwe, where the rate for only one hospital is recorded. However, the frequency of cesarean sections rose more quickly in the United States than elsewhere. By 1980, the U.S. rate had soared above most of the 15 other countries for which data are available. The only possible exception was Brazil, where middle- and upper-class urban women may face the highest probability in the world of delivering by cesarean section. Canada followed closely behind the United States, with Finland, Scotland, and Sweden clustered together next. Zaire, Czechoslovakia, the Netherlands, India, and Saudi Arabia had the lowest rates. As of 1985, the most recent year for which data from many countries are available, the picture had not changed much. More-detailed Australian data for 1986 (Renwick, 1991), however, show an interesting phenomenon. Although the national average remained lower than in the United States, the range among mainland states and territories (15.1 to 26.3 percent) and the coefficient of variation (.20) were similar to those of the American states (reported in Table 5).

Four main diagnoses account for the majority of cesarean sections in the United States. They are previous cesarean, breech presentation, fetal distress, and dystocia. Cesareans related to these diagnoses in the United States and Canada are treated more thoroughly later in this report. For purposes of comparison with those rates in the United States, the rates of cesarean section among women assigned these four diagnoses are presented in Table 2. These rates should be interpreted

Table 2

International Cesarean Rates for Given Diagnoses

Country	Ref	Year	Previous Cesarean	Breech	Fetal Distress	Dystocia
Australia, South	J1	1986		91.4	32.4	
Australia, Tasmania	M9	1975		3.3	8.4	33.9
	M9	1976		5.2	11.6	31.8
	M9	1977		12.8	13.0	34.0
	M9	1978		11.9	13.4	31.0
	M9	1979		14.4	12.1	29.4
	M9	1980		16.4	10.1	34.0
	M9	1981		18.4	14.3	35.1
	M9	1982		25.4	14.0	33.3
Bavaria	N3	1980	66.7	67.1	27.3	
	N3	1985	61.0	79.8	37.9	
Canada	N3	1980	96.2	55.0	24.3	
	L2	1980	96	55		
	N3	1984	94.3	69.2	24.2	
Colombia†	L3	1977		34.3		
Denmark	N3	1979		55.8		
	N3	1983		75.4	21.6	
England & Wales	L2	1980		76		
Hungary	N3	1980	67.4	32.7	25.5	
	N3	1983		38.7	27.0	
	N3	1985	68.3			
India, 1 Calcutta hospital	D1	1980-81	25.1			
Italy, Latium region	B3	1985		71.8		
Netherlands	N3	1980	41.1	24.5	18.8	
	N3	1985	44.6	34.8	21.5	
New Zealand	N3	1982	87.7	41.5	29.5	
	L1	1983-84				15.2
	N3	1985	81.8	45.9	29.8	
Norway	N3	1980	57.4			
	L2	1980	57	45		
	N3	1983	53.5			
Scotland	N3	1980	61.3			
	N3	1982	60.7			
	L2	1982	97	67		
Sweden	N3	1980		91.9		
	L2	1981	93			
	N3	1985		93.3		

Table 2--continued

Country	Source	Year	Previous Cesarean	Breech	Fetal Distress	Dystocia
US	S2	1970	98.3	11.6		50.6
	S2	1974	98.5	26.7	60.1	59.6
	S2	1978	98.9	60.1	59.0	67.0
	S3	1979	98.7*			
	T2	1980	96.6	66.2	62.8	66.7
	N3	1980			66.9	
	P2,P3	1981	96.4			
	P2,P3	1982	95.2			
	P2,P3	1983	95.4			
	S2	1984	96.1	79.8	31.9	65.7
	S3	1984	95.2*			
	P2,P3	1984	94.3			
	P2,P3,T2,V2	1985	93.4	79.1	45.6	65.2
	N3	1985			55.7	
	P2,P3,V2	1986	91.5			
	V2	1987	90.2			
	V2	1988	87.4			
	V2	1989	81.5	80.6*	33.3*	59.5*
	V2	1990	79.6			

* Inferred from data presented by source and subject to a rounding error.
† Data represent a sample of urban hospitals between March and October 1977.

NOTE: Please round all of the numbers in this table to the nearest whole percentage point.

only generally; it is likely that in different places slightly different criteria are used to assign diagnoses. Nevertheless, it appears that there is substantial variation in the treatment given in response to the diagnoses.

Previous cesarean is the most clear-cut of the four conditions. Little variation ought to exist in assigning this diagnosis. The repeat cesarean rate was between 90 and 100 percent in the United States, Canada, and Sweden in 1980. The percentage given repeat cesareans was in the 60s in Bavaria, Hungary, and Scotland; in the 50s in Norway; and in the 40s in the Netherlands. In India, three-quarters of women with previous cesareans delivered vaginally. The U.S. cesarean rate for the other three diagnoses is, with few exceptions, again the highest.

Were cesareans performed according to medical need alone, we would expect to find the highest rates in places where prenatal care is likely to be inadequate by current standards. In this case, we would expect developing countries to have higher rates than developed ones. Very low rates in Zaire, Saudi Arabia, and Czechoslovakia, coupled with high rates in the United States and Canada, belie this hypothesis. Alternatively, we might expect that since cesarean sections require a costly medical facility and highly trained doctors, cesarean rates would be lower in less-developed nations. However, the strikingly frequent use of cesarean section in Brazil and Puerto Rico, and the rarity of the procedure in the Netherlands, Japan, Switzerland, and Sweden, argue against this view.

Both these factors--medical need and financial wherewithal--surely affect the frequency with which cesareans are performed. Yet the interplay between these and other factors makes cesarean rates unpredictable. What is clear from these data is great disproportion; while many women suffer unnecessary cesareans, many others lack access to an operation that may save their children's or their own lives.

LARGE AREA VARIATIONS IN THE UNITED STATES AND CANADA

The tables presented in this section show total C-section rates as reported in the literature by geographic location within the United States (and Canada, since the rates are so similar) for each year from 1970 to 1990. Again, each line in the tables represents data from one source.

The most striking feature of the total U.S. cesarean rate is its monotonic increase from 1970 to 1988. A complete set of figures from 1970 until 1990, based on the National Hospital Discharge Survey, is shown on the first line of Table 3. Data provided by several references (P2, P3, T1, and T2) show a steady increase through 1987, more than quadrupling from 5.5 percent in 1970 to 24.4 percent in 1987. VanTuinen and Wolfe (V2) report the first decline in the cesarean rate in two decades, from a high of 24.7 in 1988 to 23.8 in 1989 and 23.5 in 1990. Canadian rates followed a remarkably similar pattern, at least until 1982, although they seem to trail those in the United States slightly.

Table 3

Total Cesarean Section Rates, by Year and Geographic Area, U.S. and Regional Data Only

Region	Ref	1970	1971	1972	1973	1974	1975	1976	1977	1978	1979	1980	1981	1982	1983	1984	1985	1986	1987	1988	1989	1990
US	N4,P2,P3,T1,T2,V2	5.5	5.8	7.0	8.0	9.2	10.4	12.1	13.7	15.2	16.4	16.5	17.9	18.5	20.3	21.1	22.7	24.1	24.4	24.7	23.8	23.5
	S2	5.7				9.2				14.7						21.2						
	S3										14.1					19.0						
	N3																23					
Midwest	M3,P2,P5,T1	4.7	5.2	5.7	7.0	8.4	9.3	10.6		13.9		14.9			18.8	18.9		23.2	23.2			
	S3															17.1						
North East	M3,P2,P5,T1	6.2	7.4	7.3	9.0	10.8	11.9	14.6		17.6		19.2			21.5	21.4		25.4	26.4			
	S3															20.2						
South	M3,P2,P5,T1	5.8	5.2	7.4	8.0	9.3	10.5	12.1		15.2		16.8			21.3	22.7		24.8	25.5			
	S3															20.4						
West	M3,P2,P5,T1	5.7	5.7	8.3	8.0	8.1	9.9	11.3		14.6		15.3			19.1	20.6		22.9	22.5			
	S3															18.9						
Canada	N4,W1	5.7	6.4	7.2	8.0	9.0	9.6	10.8	12.1	13.9	15.1	15.9	17.0	18.3								
	L2	6.0	6.4	7.2	8.0	9.0	9.6	10.8	12.1	13.9	14.7	15.2	15.8									
	N3															[	19	]				

Zahniser et al. (1992) report that the 48 percent rise in C-sections between 1980 and 1987 (from an estimated 617,000 procedures to 949,000) was accompanied by a 43 percent decline in forceps deliveries (from 539,000 to 320,000) and a 450 percent increase in vacuum deliveries (from 22,000 to 122,000).

Cesarean rates by region mirror the national pattern of increase (see Table 3). Women in every part of the country stood a greater chance of delivering by C-section in each succeeding year until 1986. However, the rate of cesarean differed in absolute terms across regions. The difference between the highest and the lowest regional rate was a minimum of 2.0 percent (in 1973) and a maximum of 4.3 percent (in 1980). Over 19 percent of birthing women in the Northeast had cesareans in 1980, while only 14.9 percent of Midwestern women did. The Northeastern rate was almost 30 percent higher than the Midwestern rate that year. In fact, the Northeast was consistently above the national average and had the highest rate in almost every year for which we have data. (1972 was the exception.) And the Midwest was the only region consistently below the national average, having the lowest rate in every year but 1974. The West was above average in 1970 and 1972 but has been below it since. It actually had the lowest rates of all the regions in 1986 and 1987 and was the only region to show an absolute decline during those years. The South has remained either above or right at the national average with the exception of 1971. As of 1987, the last year for which we have data, the Northeast had the highest rate, followed by the South, the Midwest, and the West with the lowest rate.

Rates by state (Table 4) showed a greater spread than by region, as would be expected. Nevertheless, the rates were surprisingly uniform in terms of their steady increase. In fact, only three states (Massachusetts, Georgia, and Pennsylvania) had lower rates for a year or two during the 1970s or early 1980s before resuming an upward trajectory. Seven states (Arizona, Colorado, Maryland, Massachusetts, Missouri, Rhode Island, and Washington) led the recent national decline by lowering their cesarean rates between 1986 and 1988.

Table 4

Total Cesarean Section Rates, by Year and Geographic Area, States Only

State	Ref	1970	1971	1972	1973	1974	1975	1976	1977	1978	1979	1980	1981	1982	1983	1984	1985	1986	1987	1988	1989	1990
AL	S4,V2•																		17.9		25.7	25.9
AK	V2																				15.2	15.3
AZ	S4,V2•																		22.2	20.8		19.9
AR	S4,V2•																		24.3		27.1	27.8
CA	S9	6.9	7.6	8.7	9.9	11.3	12.8	14.0	15.4	15.7	16.5	17.1	17.3	18.5	20.0	20.8	21.6	23.1				
CA	W5	6.9	7.6	8.7	9.9	11.3	12.8	14.0	15.4													
CA	G1,G2								15	16	16	17	17	18.4								
CA	S7														21.7	22.6	23.2	24.5	25.0			
CA	W6															20.9	21.7	23.1	23.6	22.9		
CA	P6	6.9					12.8					17.1			19.8							
CA	P1						12.7															
CA	V2																				22.9	21.4
CO	S4																	20.6	20.2			
CT	P6											18.7			20.7							
CT	S4,V2•																	23.2	24.6			21.9
DE	V2																				26.6	25.3
DC	G1,G2								19	20	22	24	24	27	27.2							
DC	S4,V2•																	30.1	30.3		25.0	26.6
FL	S4,V2•																24.8	27.7	27.9			26.4
GA	G1,G2								13.2	15.6	13.5	15.5	15.9	19.3	19.6							
GA	P6,S4,V2•											15.4			19.9				24.9		23.2	22.3
HI	S4,V2•																			22.8		20.6
ID	V2																					18.9
IL	G1,G2									14	15	16	17	18	18.7							
IL	S4,V2•																	22.3			21.9	
IN	S4,V2•																	21			21.2	
IA	S4,V2•																		20.9			18.9
KS	P6	4.3					9.0					16.1			20.7							
KS	S4,V2•																	26.5	27.4		23.7	23.4
KY	V2																				23.6	23.8
LA	V2																					27.3
ME	P6														17.9							
ME	S4,V2•																	22.1	23.1			22.2

Table 4--continued

State	Ref	1970	1971	1972	1973	1974	1975	1976	1977	1978	1979	1980	1981	1982	1983	1984	1985	1986	1987	1988	1989	1990
MD*	P6	5.7					12.8					20.6			23.6							
MD	S4,V2•																	26.6	26.4	26.0		24.4
MA	M2							13.9	15.3	17.7	19.0	19.0	19.5	20.1								
MA	G1,G2								15.3	17.7	19.0	18.4	19.5	19.4	20.1							
MA	M1																		24.6	24.4		
MA	S4,V2•																	23.7			22.9	
MI	G1,G2										9.0	10.0	10.8	11.7	12.7							
MI	S4,V2•																	25			22.9	22.0
MN	P6	4.3					7.9					13.9			16.3							
MN	S4,V2•																	17.2	19		18.1	17.6
MS	S4,V2•																		26.2			26.3
MO	P6	4.7					9.2					15.1			19.0							
MO	M5			6.0									16.1									
MO	G1,G2									13.2	14.1	14.8	15.8	17.3	18.6							
MO	S4,V2•																		24.7	24.5		23.3
MT	P6	5.0					7.4					12.6			15.5							
MT	S4,V2•																		19.7		20.7	20.9
NE	G6,G7	5.5	5.7	5.8	7	7.4	8.3	9.6	10.4	11.8	13.1	13.5		15								
NE	V2																					19.6
NV	S4,V2•																		19.2		31.7	
NH	P6									15.0					19.6							
NH	S4,V2•																	23.0	23.3		22.0	22.2†
NJ	H1	6.1	6.8	7.5	8.7	9.9	10.1	13.5	15.1	16.6	18.1	19.5	20.2	21.4	22.0	23.9	24.8	26.7				
NJ	S4,V2•																	26.8			27.0	
NM	P6											14.7			17.2							
NM	S4,V2•																		20		18.7	18.5
NY	G1,G2								14	16	17	18	19	20.7	20.8							
NY	S4,V2•																24.2	25.8			23.5	23.6
NC	S4,V2•																			24		23.0
ND	S4,V2•																		19.8			19.3
OH	S4,V2•																	23.9			25.9	25.7
OR	S4,V2•																		22.4		21.0	
PA	G1,G2								12	9	15	16	17	17.8	18.9							
PA	P6	5.6					10.0					16.0			19.3							
PA	S4,V2•																	22.7	23.9		23.0	21.9

Table 4--continued

State	Ref	1970	1971	1972	1973	1974	1975	1976	1977	1978	1979	1980	1981	1982	1983	1984	1985	1986	1987	1988	1989	1990
RI	H3																	23.8	23.1	22.4		
RI	V2																				20.8	20.0
SC	S4,V2•																		23.7			22.8§
TN	S4,V2•																	20.4	20.8		24.4	24.5
TX	V2																				25.9	
UT	P6									10.1		11.7			13.9							
UT	S4,V2•																	18			18.4	17.9
VT	P6									13.8		15.0			17.2							
VT	S4,V2•																		20.1		19.1	19.4
VA	G1,G2										9.3	9.3	13.7	15.0	15.9							
VA	S4,V2•																	19.1	19.2		24.1†	24.1
WA	P6											14.3			16.5							
WA	S4,V2•																		21.9	21.7		21.0†
WV	S4,V2•																		24.6		25.4	26.3
WI	N1	5.0	5.4	5.8	6.6	7.5	8.2	9.3	10.4													
WI	K1	5.0	5.4	5.9	6.7	7.6	8.3	9.5	10.6	12.1	12.9	13.6	14.3	15.2	15.8	17.4	17.9					
WI	S4,V2•																	19.2			17.5	17.5
WY	S4,V2•																[18.5	]	[21.2	]	18.5	19.6

* Data represent births ocurring to all residents of Maryland regardless of state of delivery.

† Indicates data for a six-month period.

§ Data for 1990 fiscal year.

• 1986 and 1987 rates are from reference S4. 1989 and 1990 rates are from reference V2.

Geographic variation exists, but how important is it? Our data are most complete for 1987, followed by 1986, 1983, and 1980. For 1987, we have figures for 32 of 50 states plus Washington, D.C.; unless by coincidence we have data for the states with the highest and lowest cesarean rates, our data understate the true spread. Nonetheless, they are adequate to make the point that state-to-state variation is considerable. In 1987, the difference between the highest and the lowest state rate was at least 12.4 percent; Alabama had a low rate of 17.9 percent, while 30.3 percent of women in Washington, D.C., were delivering by cesarean. If we exclude Washington, D.C., the difference was still a full 10 percent. (The next highest rate was in Florida at 27.9 percent). 1979, 1980, 1986, and 1987 all show spreads of at least 10 percent (see Table 5), and in 1979 and 1980, the highest rate is over twice the lowest.

Table 5

The Size of Variations in Cesarean Section Rates Among States

Year	N	Range	Coeff of Var
1970	10	4.3 to 6.9	0.15
1971	4	5.4 to 7.6	0.14
1972	5	5.5 to 8.7	0.17
1973	4	6.7 to 9.9	0.16
1974	4	7.4 to 11.3	0.18
1975	10	7.4 to 12.8	0.19
1976	5	9.5 to 14.0	0.17
1977	8	10.4 to 15.4	0.15
1978	13	9.0 to 17.7	0.18
1979	12	9.0 to 19.0	0.21
1980	21	9.3 to 19.5	0.19
1981	11	10.8 to 20.2	0.16
1982	12	11.7 to 21.4	0.15
1983	22	12.7 to 22.0	0.14
1984	3	17.4 to 23.9	0.13
1985	6	17.9 to 24.8	0.13
1986	24	17.2 to 30.1	0.14
1987	32	17.9 to 30.3	0.13
1988	10	20.8 to 26.0	0.07

Coefficients of variation were typically around 15-20 percent. Chassin et al. (1986) calculated coefficients of variation for over one hundred procedures used by Medicare patients in 13 large areas of the United States (states or large portions of states) and divided the procedures into three groups based on the amount of variation. A coefficient of variation of 15-20 percent would put cesareans into the group of procedures with the least variation from area to area.

Caution must be exercised in comparing state and regional data from different sources. We would expect about half the states to have higher, and half lower, cesarean rates than the averages reported for their respective regions. However, almost all the state figures are lower than their regional averages. Since we have at least one datum for most states, it is unlikely that we have collected all the low rates and are missing all the high ones. It is more probable that either the regional or some of the state data (or both) reflect a systematic bias that makes them incomparable. Nevertheless, we should still be able to roughly rank states or regions, particularly when using data from the same source. We should also be able to trust the temporal pattern of changing rates within the same area. Note also that the ranges presented in Table 5 should not be interpreted as a time series since different states are represented in different years.

SMALL AREA VARIATIONS IN THE UNITED STATES

City and county rates, although sparse, are interesting for two reasons (see Table 6). First, we might expect urban areas to be either consistently higher or consistently lower than their respective state rates, but such a pattern does not appear to exist. Women in Boston, New York City, and Philadelphia County deliver by cesarean at a higher rate than women in their states generally; but in Wayne County (which includes Detroit), St. Louis, Atlanta, Sacramento, and San Francisco, women are less likely to have C-sections. Cesarean rates in Los Angeles, San Diego, and Chicago are much the same as the state rates. We cannot expect, therefore, that urban hospitals are the cause, or will be the cure, for the general cesarean section problem.

Second, the rates reported for Massachusetts towns and California counties show that medical practice is not uniform even within fairly small geographical areas. The California counties included in Table 6 were selected on the basis of size; they are the 12 counties with the largest number of births in 1989. The difference between the highest and the lowest of these county rates is at least 4 percent in each year. The Massachusetts town rates were selected not by number of births, but to illustrate variation. Acker et al. (1988, A1) present cesarean rates for towns with significantly high and significantly low ratios of actual to expected cesarean rates after controlling for differences in maternal age. The 30.4 percent cesarean rate in Winthrop is well over twice the 13.5 percent rate in North Adams. Random variation could account for a substantial portion of the spread among the smaller cities in the table. To illustrate, Winthrop is the smallest; its rate is based on only 181 deliveries, so a 95 percent confidence interval around its rate of 30.4 percent is 23.1 to 37.1.

VARIATIONS BY HOSPITAL AND PHYSICIAN

There are a handful of studies that report the distribution of C-section rates across some group of hospitals or physicians (see Table 7). They generally show a fairly substantial amount of variation, comparable to that reported by Chassin et al. (1986) for "moderately" or "highly" varying medical and surgical services across 13 large areas of the United States. One is not surprised to find more variation among smaller units (hospitals or physicians, rather than states).

CONCLUSION

The dramatic variations in C-section rates make it clear that more than strict medical need influences the decision to perform a C-section.

The rest of the report will attempt to identify explanatory variables and explain their relative importance. Variables that affect the decision to perform a C-section fall into two general categories. On one hand, variations in the interpretation of clinical conditions coupled with variations in methods of dealing with those conditions have large effects on cesarean rates. These issues will be considered next in the "clinical" section of this report. On the other hand, the

Table 6

Total Cesarean Section Rates, by Year and Geographic Area, City and County Data Only

Area	Ref	1970...	1975...	1977	1978	1979	1980	1981	1982	1983	1984	1985	1986	1987	1988
Los Angeles Cty, CA	A1,G2			15	16	16	17	17	18.3						
Los Angeles Cty, CA	P6										21.0	21.7	22.9	24.5	24.1
San Diego Cty, CA	P6										20.2	22.3	23.9	22.1	21.9
Orange Cty, CA	P6										23.7	24.1	25.7	25.4	24.3
Santa Clara Cty, CA	P6										18.7	20.7	21.2	21.7	20.1
San Bernardino Cty, CA	P6										21.2	21.3	23.6	23.9	23.3
Alameda Cty, CA	P6										20.7	21.9	22.1	22.2	21.3
Riverside Cty, CA	P6										21.6	22.0	23.2	23.6	23.2
Sacramento Cty, CA	P6										18.6	18.4	20.6	20.6	20.8
Contra Costa Cty, CA	P6										25.9	25.8	26.7	26.2	24.4
San Francisco Cty, CA	P6										19.7	19.5	20.8	21.7	21.9
Ventura Cty, CA	P6										22.5	23.1	24.6	24.7	23.3
Fresno Cty, CA	P6										22.0	22.5	23.8	23.5	23.9
Chicago, IL	A1,G2				14	15	16	17	18	18.7					
St. Louis, MO	A1,G2				12.9	13.2	13.4	13.9	16.3	16.8					
Wayne Cty-Detroit, MI	A1,G2						9.9	10.8	11.4	12.3					
Greater Boston, MA	A1,G2			19.5	20.8	22.4	22.1	22.6	20.3	20.3					
Winthrop MA	A1											30.4			
Attleboro MA	A1											28.3			
Milton MA	A1											30.1			
Braintree MA	A1											28.0			
Quincy MA	A1											27.2			
Lynn MA	A1											26.2			
Weymouth MA	A1											26.1			
Springfield MA	A1											24.2			
Webster MA	A1											17.5			
Andover MA	A1											18.1			
Fairhaven MA	A1											16.3			
Littleboro MA	A1											16.4			
Millbury MA	A1											14.4			
North Adams MA	A1											13.5			
NY City, NY	P6	5.0	8.3		19.1					20.4					
NY City, NY	A1,G2				19	20	20	21	22	20.3					
Upstate NY	P6	5.7	10.3				18.9			21.8					
Philadelphia Cty, PA	A1,G2			14	9	16	17	18	18.8	20.6					
Atlanta, GA	A1,G2			10.7	12.4	13.0	14.1	15.2	17.8	21.8					
New Orleans, LA	W2											28.2			
Washington DC	A1,G2			19	20	22	24	24	27	27.2					

Table 7

Variations by Hospital, Physician, or Zip Code

Reference	Range	Coefficient of variation
Halpin, Rose & Shapiro 1989, H1: 1986, New Jersey, primary C-sections;71 hospitals	8.7 to 31.1	0.24
DeMott & Sandmire 1990, D3: 1986-88, Green Bay, WI, C-sections for singleton delivery; 11 physicians	5.6 to 19.7	0.30
Adams 1983, A2: 1977-79, southeastern MN, C-sections for low-risk women; 15 hospitals	0.0 to 10.4	0.64
Zdeb, Therriault & Logrillo 1980, Z3: 1977-78, upstate NY, primary C-sections; 151 hospitals	1.1 to 22.5	0.48
Zdeb, Therriault & Logrillo 1989, Z2: 1984-86, New York State, overall C-sections; all hospitals in NYS	11.1 to 43.8	na
Zdeb, Therriault & Logrillo 1989, Z2: 1984-86, New York State, primary C-sections; all hospitals in NYS	7.3 to 32.5	na
Zdeb, Therriault & Logrillo 1989, Z2: 1984-86, New York State, secondary C-sections; all hospitals in NYS	3.0 to 16.1	na
Zdeb, Therriault & Logrillo 1989, Z2: 1984-86, New York State, overall C-sections; 2126 physicians with at least 60 deliveries	under 10.0 included 9% 20.0 to 30.0 included 85% 40.0 and over included 0.3%	
Zdeb, Therriault & Logrillo 1989, Z2: 1984-86, New York State, overall C-sections; 968 zip codes with at least 50 live births	8.5 to 40.1	na
Williams & Wroblewski 1991, W6: 1984-88, California, overall C-sections; all facilities with at least one birth each year	percentiles 10th 90th 14.3 to 30.8	na

NOTE: na denotes not available.

"nonclinical" section addresses the effect of nonmedical characteristics, such as the patient's socioeconomic status, whether the patient has medical insurance, and the type of physician practice.

3. VARIATIONS AMONG MAJOR DIAGNOSES AFFECTING CESAREAN RATES

Regardless of the influence of nonclinical factors, all cesareans are attributed to a medical condition. Four such conditions jointly account for the overwhelming, and increasing, majority of cesarean sections. Estimates vary slightly, but the most recent data show that as of 1987 previous cesarean, dystocia, fetal distress, and breech presentation accounted for 83 percent of all cesareans (Taffel, 1989). In 1980, they accounted for only 77 percent. This report addresses the four diagnoses in detail. Remaining cesareans are attributed to a multitude of less frequent complications--placenta previa, for example, or diabetes. (For a dated but manageable list of such additional complications, see Placek and Taffel, 1983). These less-frequent diagnoses are not generally considered to be a logical focus of efforts to reduce cesarean rates, both because their potential contribution is so small and because of the wide agreement concerning the gravity of many of the problems.

There are two major components to the contribution to C-section rates of a diagnosis. First, how frequently is the diagnosis made? Second, how frequently is a C-section used to treat the diagnosis? Changes in either of these components over time have repercussions for total cesarean rates. The two factors can move in the same direction, each reinforcing the effect of the other, or they can move in opposite directions, one canceling out the other effect. In Tables 9 through 12, the first two lines associated with each data source show these two sets of figures. The first line, "% with diagnosis," shows the percentage of all birthing women assigned the diagnosis in question. The second line, "% with c-sec," indicates the percentage of all similarly diagnosed women who were given C-sections. To understand the overall importance of these rates, we need two more configurations of the information. The third line shows the percentage of all cesareans that are performed in response to the given diagnosis. The fourth line shows the percentage of the total population of birthing women who were given C-sections for the diagnosis. To reduce the cesarean section rate, this fourth line must decline over time. As of 1989, the last year for which we have data, such a decline had not taken place for any of the diagnoses. Therefore, we cannot be sure of the origin of the recent decline in the total U.S. cesarean rate.

Many of the figures were taken directly from the articles referenced. Others were calculated secondhand on the basis of data in the articles and are marked with an asterisk. For example, "% of total births" can be calculated by multiplying "% with diagnosis" by "% with C-sec" and dividing by 100. And "% of all C-sec" equals "% of total births" divided by the total cesarean rate as given by the same source times 100.

Data for diagnoses are not as complete as for overall rates, so analyzing geographic variations in rates by diagnoses is not possible. However, given the wide variety of overall rates, it cannot be assumed that physicians in different areas treat similar indications in the same way. We cannot even assume that high cesarean rates in two states are being driven by the same forces. More diagnosis-specific data analysis by area must be done to most effectively target efforts at cesarean reduction.

PREVIOUS C-SECTION

The dictum "once a cesarean always a cesarean" has done much to boost the total cesarean rate. Primary C-sections increased monotonically from 4.2 percent of births to women with no previous cesarean in 1970, to 17.5 percent of such births in 1986 (see Table 8). Since then the rate has dropped to 16.8 percent in 1990. This means that even with a stable rate of vaginal birth after cesarean (VBAC), we would begin to see decreases in the proportion of all birthing women who are given repeat cesareans without other medical indications. However, the second line of Table 9 shows that VBAC has become more common as well. Although data are sparse, the figures corresponding to "% with diagnosis" (see Table 9) show that the proportion of women with previous cesareans has been rising steadily in every location for which we have data. This increase results from the rising rate of primary cesareans for other diagnoses.

Table 8

Primary Cesareans

Year	Primary Cesareans
1970	4.2
1975	7.8
1980	12.1
1981	12.5
1982	13.3
1983	14.3
1984	15.0
1985	16.0
1986	17.4
1987	17.4
1988	17.5
1989	17.1
1990	16.8

Source: 1980-1987, Taffel 1989; 1988-1990, VanTuinen and Wolfe, 1992.

Trials of labor after previous cesareans used to be discouraged primarily for fear that the old uterine scar would rupture during labor. The concern was valid for classical, vertical incisions. However, the popularity of such incisions waned many years ago in favor of lower transverse incisions, which are significantly stronger and come under less stress during labor (Miller and Sutter, 1985). During the 1980s, physicians began conducting controlled trials of labor among women with previous cesareans. Reviews by Miller and Sutter (1985), Shiono et al. (1987), and Haq (1988) cite studies that show between 51 percent and 89 percent success rates for attempted VBAC. They also show no maternal deaths, and few or no fetal deaths due to uterine rupture. Physicians seem to be responding to this new information; rates of repeat cesareans are decreasing everywhere. Nationwide rates have dropped from 93.4 percent in 1985 to 81.5 percent in 1990 by one measure.

Repeat cesareans as a percentage of all cesareans seem to have been hovering between 30 percent and 36 percent, nationally, although in some states the figure is higher. Using 1989 rates, if trials of labor could be conducted in all cases of previous cesarean, and if only the lower-

Table 9

Repeat Cesarean Section Rates, by Year and Geographic Area

Area	Ref		1970	1971	1972	1973	1974	1975	1976	1977	1978	1979	1980	1981	1982	1983	1984	1985	1986	1987	1988	1989	1990
US	S2	% with diagnosis	2.1				2.8				4.6						7.9						
		% with c-sec	98.3				98.5				98.9						96.1						
		% of all c-secs	36.8*				30.4*				30.6*						36.0						
		% of total births	2.1*				2.8*				4.5*						7.6*						
US	P2,P3,	% with diagnosis											5.1					8.4		7.8*		10.4*	
	T1,T2,	% with c-sec											96.6	96.4	95.2	95.4	94.3	93.4	91.5	90.2	87.4	81.5	79.6
	V2	% of all c-secs	25.2					27.1					29.9	34.3	32.2	34.8	34.2	34.6	34.3	35.3		35.6	
		"											29.7					34.8					
		% of total births	1.4*					2.8*					4.9	6.1*	5.9*	7.1*	7.2*	7.9	8.3*	8.6*		8.5*	
US	S3	% with diagnosis																					
		% with c-sec										98.7*					95.2*						
		% of all c-secs																					
		% of total births																					
Northeast	T1	% of total births											5*								7.9*		
Midwest		% of total births											3.6*								6.9*		
South		% of total births											4.5*								7.0*		
West		% of total births											4.4*								6.2*		
Ontario	A5	% with diagnosis										5.8			7.6	8.1		8.6		8.8			
		% with c-sec										97.7			95.2	95.0		94.3		91.3			
		% of all c-secs										34.5			38.5	39.1		40.1		39.9			
		% of total births										5.7			7.2	7.7		8.1		8.1			
CA	S7,S8	% with diagnosis														8.6	9.1	9.2	9.9	10.2			
		% with c-sec														93.0	91.4	89.9	89.2	87.4			
		% of all c-secs														36.9*	36.7*	35.8*	35.7	35.6*			
		% of total births														8.0*	8.3*	8.3*	8.8*	8.9*			
CA	W6	% with diagnosis																					
		% with c-sec																					
		% of all c-secs															36.4*	35.5*	35.5*	35.2*	36.7*		
		% of total births															7.6	7.7	8.2	8.3	8.4		
CA **	S9	% with diagnosis																	9.7				
		% with c-sec																	89.2				
		% of all c-secs																	35.8				
		% of total births																	8.7*				

Table 9--continued

Area	Ref		1970	1971	1972	1973	1974	1975	1976	1977	1978	1979	1980	1981	1982	1983	1984	1985	1986	1987	1988	1989	1990
CT	P6	% with diagnosis																					
		% with c-sec																					
		% of all c-secs														37.7							
		% of total births														20.7							
GA	P6	% with diagnosis																					
		% with c-sec																					
		% of all c-secs														34.4							
		% of total births														19.9							
MA	M1	% with diagnosis																					
		% with c-sec																					
		% of all c-secs																		37.5	37.5		
		% of total births																		9.0	9.1		
NE	G6,G7	% with diagnosis																					
		% with c-sec																					
		% of all c-secs	38.2*	38.6*	37.9*	34.3*	32.4*	32.5*	32.3*	32.7*	33.1*				43.3*								
		% of total births	2.1	2.2	2.2	2.4	2.4	2.7	3.1	3.4	3.9				6.5								
RI	H3	% with diagnosis																					
		% with c-sec																		86.0	83.0		
		% of all c-secs																			40.2*		
		% of total births																			9.0		
UT	P6	% with diagnosis																					
		% with c-sec																					
		% of all c-secs														42.1							
		% of total births														13.9							
WA	P6	% with diagnosis																					
		% with c-sec																					
		% of all c-secs														37.7							
		% of total births														16.5							

% with diagnosis - number of women diagnosed as having a previous c-section divided by the total number of births.

% with c-sec - number of women given a repeat c-section divided by the number with diagnosis.

% of all c-secs - number of women with a repeat c-section divided by the total number of c-sections.

% of total births - number of women given a repeat cesarean section divided by the total number of births.

* Inferred from data presented by source and subject to a rounding error.

** Data are based on January through June only.

bound 50 percent success rate held good, the proportion of the total population having cesareans could be reduced by 4.25 percent. Such a goal is probably unrealistic, however. First, women with other complications may not be good candidates for a trial of labor. Second, due to the small but real possibility of uterine rupture, American College of Obstetricians and Gynecologists (ACOG) guidelines recommend that trials be conducted only when an emergency staff is on duty, with constant attendance by an anesthesiologist, and only when preparation for an emergency cesarean can be completed within 30 minutes (Placek and Taffel, 1988). Many small hospitals do not have these capabilities around the clock and cannot offer trials of labor at night. However, there is certainly room for improvement among larger hospitals, some of which do not offer trials despite the availability of the required services (Haq, 1988). As of 1984, only 54 percent of all hospitals offered trials of labor. For small hospitals the percentage was much lower, but even among large hospitals, 30 percent did not accept trials (Shiono et al., 1987, S3). Although these figures are old, it would appear that increasing the incidence of VBAC is a feasible way to lower the cesarean rate.

BREECH PRESENTATION

Though only a small percentage of babies are breech, the rate of breech presentation appears to be dropping slightly in the United States due to an increase in successful external cephalic version (see Table 10). One source shows a large drop from 2.9 percent in 1970 to 2.3 percent in 1984 (Shiono et al., 1987, S2). Another shows a smaller decrease from 3.1 percent to 2.9 percent between 1980 and 1985 (Taffel, 1989, T1). However, the California rate has held fairly constant from 1983 to 1987.

In all areas for which we have data there has been a stunning rise in cesarean births for breech presentation. In 1970, less than 12 percent of breech babies in the United States were delivered by C-section. By 1989, over 80 percent were. In California, 87 percent were delivered by C-section in 1987. The cesarean rate has also risen sharply in Ontario but is still much lower than that in the United

Table 10

Cesarean Section Rates for Breech Presentations, by Year and Geographic Area

Area	Ref		1970 ...	1974 ...	1978	1979	1980	1981	1982	1983	1984	1985	1986	1987	1988	1989
US	S2	% with diagnosis	2.9	2.7	2.8						2.3					
		% with c-sec	11.6	26.7	60.1						79.8					
		% of all c-secs	5.3*	7.6*	11.6						8.7					
		% of total births	0.3*	0.7*	1.7*						1.8*					
US	T1,T2,	% with diagnosis					3.1					2.9				3.6
	V2	% with c-sec					66.2					79.1				80.6*
		% of all c-secs					12.1					10.1		10		12.3
		% of total births					2.0					2.3				2.9
US	S3	% with diagnosis														
		% with c-sec														
		% of all c-secs				15.8					15.2					
		% of total births				2.2*					2.9*					
CA	S7,S8	% with diagnosis								3.1	3.1	3.1	3.0	3.1		
		% with c-sec								81.9	82.6	85.6	86.9	87.0		
		% of all c-secs								11.5*	11.5*	11.6*	10.7	10.8*		
		% of total births								2.5*	2.6*	2.7*	2.6*	2.7*		
CA **	S9	% with diagnosis											3.1			
		% with c-sec											86.6			
		% of all c-secs											10.9			
		% of total births											2.7*			
Canada	N3	% with diagnosis														
		% with c-sec					55.0					69.2				
		% of all c-secs														
		% of total births														
Ontario	A5	% with diagnosis				3.1			3.1	3.2		3.1		3.0		
		% with c-sec				54.8			65.0	64.7		68.2		68.1		
		% of all c-secs				10.3			10.7	10.5		10.6		10.2		
		% of total births				1.7			2.0	2.1		2.1		2.1		

% with diagnosis - number of women diagnosed as having a breech presentation divided by the total number of births.
% with c-sec - number of women given a c-section due to breech presentation divided by the number with diagnosis.
% of all c-secs - number of women given a c-section due to breech presentation divided by the total number of c-sections.
% of total births - number of women given a c-section due to breech presentation divided by the total number of births.
* Inferred from data presented by source and subject to a rounding error.
** Data are based on January through June only.

States. Some studies have attributed the increase to the fact that young doctors are no longer being trained to deliver breech babies vaginally (Anderson and Lomas, 1984).

Cesarean sections due to breech presentation are becoming more common in the total population. There is no medical reason why certain types of breech cannot be delivered vaginally, so reemphasizing the legitimacy of vaginal deliveries in some cases and encouraging training in the proper techniques could be a valuable endeavor. However, given the low incidence of breech presentation, modifying physician behavior for this diagnosis does not have the same potential payoff as increasing VBAC rates.

DYSTOCIA

Dystocia, like previous cesarean, is a large contributor to the overall cesarean rate (see Table 11). Its incidence has risen in the United States, California, and Ontario--the only places for which we have data. In fact, the rate of diagnosis of dystocia in the United States rose from 3.8 percent in 1970 (Shiono, et al., 1987, S2) to 11.6 percent in 1989 (VanTuinen and Wolfe, 1992, V2). The reasons for the rising incidence of dystocia are less clear than for previous cesarean, however. Dystocia is a catch-all diagnosis for difficult labor, long labor, failure to progress, and even cephalopelvic disproportion. It is to a large extent a question of physician judgment. There is some feeling that doctors are increasingly treating average labor as expected labor, and anything longer or more difficult as abnormal (Sheehan, 1987; Stewart et al., 1990). There is also speculation that the increasing incidence of dystocia is the result of physicians' unwillingness to allow long labor, at least in part for fear of the malpractice potential inherent in any bad fetal outcome (Sheehan, 1987).

A slight drop in the rate of C-sections in response to dystocia is counteracting some of the increase in the diagnosis of dystocia, however. The percentage with C-section is still very high in the United States, but has fallen from 67 percent in 1978 to 59.5 percent in 1989. Nevertheless, the overall effect of the two processes is that the percentage of births by cesarean due to dystocia have continued to increase, from 2.9 percent in the US in 1970 to 6.9 percent in 1989.

A unique study conducted in Ottawa, Canada, (Stewart et al., 1990) analyzed the distribution of dystocia diagnoses and cesareans by phase of labor. The authors found that 34.8 percent of the diagnoses were made in the latent phase, and more disturbingly, 41 percent of all cesareans resulting from dystocia were performed during the latent phase. (Thirty-eight percent were done during the active stage, and only 21 percent during the second stage.) These results raise questions of whether doctors allow for sufficient variation in the pattern of

Table 11

Cesarean Section Rates for Dystocia, by Year and Geographic Area

Area	Ref		1970 ...	1974 ...	1978	1979	1980	1981	1982	1983	1984	1985	1986	1987	1988	1989
US	S2	% with diagnosis	3.8	5.5	6.8						8.8					
		% with c-sec	50.6	59.6	67.0						65.7					
		% of all c-secs	33.3*	35.9*	31.2						27.5					
		% of total births	1.9*	3.3*	4.6*						5.8*					
US	T1,T2,	% with diagnosis					7.2					10.2				11.6
	V2	% with c-sec					66.7					65.2				59.5*
		% of all c-secs					29.1					29.1		28		28.9
		% of total births					4.8					6.6				6.9*
US	S3	% with diagnosis														
		% with c-sec														
		% of all c-secs				37.3					34.6					
		% of total births				5.3*					6.6*					
CA	S7,S8	% with diagnosis								11.1	11.4	11.7	12.2	12.5		
		% with c-sec								62.2	62.3	62.8	64.4	63.8		
		% of all c-secs								31.8*	31.4*	31.5*	31.9	32.0*		
		% of total births								6.9*	7.1*	7.3*	7.9*	8.0*		
CA **	S9	% with diagnosis											12.0			
		% with c-sec											64.4			
		% of all c-secs											31.8			
		% of total births											7.7*			
Ontario	A5	% with diagnosis				10.0			10.4	10.8		10.8				
		% with c-sec				33.1			32.5	31.6		32.6				
		% of all c-secs				20.0			18.2	17.4		17.3				
		% of total births				3.3			3.4	3.4		3.5				

% with diagnosis - number of women diagnosed as having dystocia divided by the total number of births.
% with c-sec - number of women given a c-section for dystocia divided by the number with diagnosis.
% of all c-secs - number of women given a c-section for dystocia divided by the total number of c-sections.
% of total births - number of women given a c-section for dystocia divided by the total number of births.
* Inferred from data presented by source and subject to a rounding error.
** Data are based on January through June only.

labor, and whether they take adequate advantage of less invasive alternatives for stimulating labor. For example, Sheehan (1987) found that more frequent oxytocin use in Ireland helped, among other factors, to keep the Irish cesarean rate for dystocia less than one-half the U.S. rate in 1980-81.

FETAL DISTRESS

The incidence of diagnosis of fetal distress has risen steeply during the 1970s and 1980s (see Table 12). By one estimate (Shiono et al., 1987, S2), it increased from 0.6 percent in 1974 to 5.8 percent in 1984 in the United States, and from 3.9 percent in 1985 to 6.3 percent in 1989 by another (VanTuinen and Wolfe, 1992, V2). In California, the incidence of fetal distress rose steadily from 5.7 percent in 1983 to

Table 12

Cesarean Section Rates Due to Fetal Distress, by Year and Geographic Area

Area	Ref		1974 ...	1978	1979	1980	1981	1982	1983	1984	1985	1986	1987	1988	1989
US	S2	% with diagnosis	0.6	1.4						5.8					
		% with c-sec	60.1	59.0						31.9					
		% of all c-secs	4.3*	5.5						8.8					
		% of total births	0.4*	0.8*						1.9*					
US	T1,T2,	% with diagnosis				1.2					3.9				6.3
	V2	% with c-sec				62.8					45.6				33.3*
		% of all c-secs				4.8					7.9		10		9.9
		% of total births				0.8					1.8				2.1*
US	S3	% with diagnosis													
		% with c-sec													
		% of all c-secs			14.4					20.5					
		% of total births			2.0*					3.9*					
US	N3	% with diagnosis													
		% with c-sec				66.9					55.7				
		% of all c-secs													
		% of total births													
CA	S7,S8	% with diagnosis							5.7	6.9	8.0	8.5	8.2		
		% with c-sec							30.2	28.9	27.8	28.5	30.6		
		% of all c-secs							7.8*	8.8*	9.5*	9.9	10.0*		
		% of total births							1.7*	2.0*	2.2*	2.4*	2.5*		
CA **	S9	% with diagnosis										8.2			
		% with c-sec										28.8			
		% of all c-secs										9.7			
		% of total births										2.4*			
Canada	N3	% with diagnosis													
		% with c-sec				24.3					24.2				
		% of all c-secs													
		% of total births													
Ontario	A5	% with diagnosis			2.4			4.7	5.4		5.8		6.4		
		% with c-sec			50.5			32.7	31.4		33.0		30.9		
		% of all c-secs			7.3			8.0	8.6		9.5		9.7		
		% of total births			1.2			1.5	1.7		1.9		1.9		

% with diagnosis - number of diagnoses of fetal distress divided by the total number of births.
% with c-sec - number of women given a c-section due to fetal distress divided by the number with diagnosis.
% of all c-secs - number of women given a c-section due to fetal distress divided by the total number of c-sections.
% of total births - number of women given a c-section due to fetal distress divided by the total number of births.
* Inferred from data presented by source and subject to rounding error.
** Data are based on January through June only.

8.2 percent in 1987 (Stafford, 1990, S7 and S8). With improvement in electronic fetal monitoring (EFM) technology, hospitals began to use EFM routinely, even in low-risk births. However, because EFM tracings may suggest the presence of problems that would not have been detected without EFM, EFM is suspected of being behind the increase in fetal distress cesareans. It is not within the scope of this report to review the separate literature on EFM and cesareans, but a fairly old review by Placek and Taffel (1980) suggests that the evidence is mixed. A later study (Taffel, Placek, and Liss, 1987) suggests that although EFM has probably increased the diagnosis of fetal distress, the jury is still out on its actual contribution to cesarean rates. A review by Monheit and Resnik (1981) indicates EFM may have generated a higher C-section rate when it was first introduced, but that as physicians gained experience with the technology, rates dropped again.

Whatever the role of EFM, physicians no longer perform C-sections in response to fetal distress diagnoses as often as they used to. The rate of C-sections due to fetal distress fell from 60.1 percent in 1974 to 31.9 percent in 1984, dropping by almost one-half within a decade. Another estimate shows an even more rapid decline of 28.6 percent between 1980 and 1985, dropping from 62.8 percent to 45.6 percent. In California, however, the downward trend has not continued in recent years. Although the California rate fell from 1983 to 1985, by 1987 it had risen again. In Canada, the rate seems to have leveled off in the 1980s after falling sharply from 1979 to 1982. It is difficult to hypothesize based on these spotty data whether we can expect to see a continued drop in the rate of cesareans for fetal distress.

Unfortunately the increase in diagnosis has more than offset the decreasing rate of diagnosis-specific C-sections. C-sections for fetal distress occur more frequently among the entire population than they used to.

CONTRIBUTIONS TO THE INCREASE IN CESAREAN RATES

Several authors have evaluated the relative contribution of the four conditions to recent increases in the total cesarean rate. The studies conclude that repeat cesareans account for between 33 percent (Shiono et al., 1987, S2) and 68 percent (Anderson and Lomas, 1984) of the increase, by far the largest share in each case. (Note that the percentages are not strictly comparable, in that the base for the Anderson and Lomas 68 percent is the increase due to the four diagnoses alone, and the base for the other studies is the total increase.) As such, it is encouraging that the most successful effort to increase vaginal delivery has been promotion of VBACs. The two U.S. studies show that dystocia takes second place, causing between 19 percent (Shiono et al., 1987, S2) and 29 percent (Taffel, et al., 1987) of the rise. While Shiono et al. (S2) conclude that breech also played a large role in the 1974 to 1978 increase; they found that by 1978 to 1984 fetal distress had overtaken breech presentation in importance. Data from 1980 to 1985 from Taffel et al. corroborate the latter finding.

Our own reanalysis of the Shiono et al. (S2) data from Tables 9 through 12 provide some additional insight into the role of the four diagnoses in the increase in C-section rates (see the last column of Table 13). The other studies all report the joint effect of change in the frequency of a diagnosis and change in the rate at which C-sections were performed for that diagnosis. We separate the two effects in our analysis. For example, over the period 1970-84, the joint effect for dystocia accounted for 25 percent of the increase in the total C-section rate. If only the frequency with which dystocia was diagnosed had increased (and the rate of C-section for dystocia had remained at the 1970 level), dystocia would have accounted for 16 percent of the increase. However, if the frequency of diagnosis of dystocia had remained the same and only the rate of C-section for dystocia had increased, dystocia would have accounted for only 4 percent of the increase. (The two components, 16 and 4 percent, do not add to the joint effect, 25 percent, because the effect of interaction between increase in diagnosis and increase in rate for diagnosis is not included.)

Our analysis shows that for previous C-section, dystocia, and fetal distress, increase in frequency of diagnosis was the more important component. For breech, the increase in the rate at which C-sections were performed was more important.

Table 13

Percentages of Contribution of Major Diagnoses to Increases in Cesarean Rates

	Anderson & Lomas 1984	Shiono, McNellis & Rhoads 1987	Shiono, McNellis & Rhoads 1987	Taffel, Placek, & Liss 1987	Heilbrunn & Park 1993*
Years	1979-82	1974-78	1978-84	1980-85	1970-84**
Where	Ontario	U.S.	U.S.	U.S.	U.S.
Previous c-section	68	32.8	46.8	48.4	35
Change in diagnosis					37
Change in rate for diagnosis					0
Breech	14	20.3***	12.4***	4.8	10
Change in diagnosis					0
Change in rate for diagnosis					13
Dystocia	4	23.4	18.9	29.0	25
Change in diagnosis					16
Change in rate for diagnosis					4
Fetal distress	14	8.5	15.8	16.1	12
Change in diagnosis					22
Change in rate for diagnosis					0
Total for four diagnoses	100	85.0	93.9	98.3	81
Other	--	15.0	6.1	1.7	19
Total	--	100.0	100.0	100.0	100

* Using data from Shiono, McNellis & Rhoads 1987
** 1974-84 for fetal distress.
*** Includes breech and other malpresentations.

4. VARIATIONS RELATED TO MATERNAL AGE AND PARITY

Two other clinical factors, in addition to physicians' diagnoses, have an effect on the overall cesarean rate: maternal age and parity. In this section, we examine studies of the temporal or geographic variation in C-section rates disaggregated by age or parity or both. Multivariate studies discussed in the following section shed some additional light on the independent effects of age and parity on C-section rates, controlling for clinical diagnoses and other factors.

MATERNAL AGE

Taffel (1989) breaks down U.S. data on total and primary cesarean sections by age for selected years from 1965 to 1987, as shown in Table 14. Two consistent patterns emerge. First, for every year studied, older women have both higher total and primary rates than women in the next youngest age group. Second, each age group experienced dramatic increases in the rate of cesarean section between 1965 and 1987. Canadian data on total cesarean rates by age from 1969 to 1976 show the same patterns (Wadhera and Nair, 1982).

In general, total cesarean rates increased faster among young women in both countries (Taffel, 1989; Wadhera and Nair, 1982). In the United States, women under 20 were six times as likely to have cesareans in 1987 as in 1965, while women over 35 were just four times as likely (Taffel, 1989). This pattern of rapid increases among young women, while true for the 22-year period as a whole, did not apply to the 1980s. Between 1980 and 1987, the rates of increase for younger age groups slowed dramatically, so that increases for older groups began to outpace them. While women under 20 were 1.3 times as likely to have cesareans in 1987 as in 1980, women over 35 were 1.5 times as likely. It appears that whatever "catching up" was done by young women occurred during the late 1960s and the 1970s.

Rates did not increase for every age category during every period, though. In fact, between 1986 and 1987, the primary cesarean rate fell for all age groups under 30, and the total rate dropped for women

Table 14

Total and Primary Cesarean Section Rates for Non-Federal Short-Stay Hospitals in the United States, by Age of Mother: Selected Years 1965 to 1987

	Age of Mother					
Year	All	Under 20	20-24	25-29	30-34	35 +
1965						
Total	4.5	3.1	3.5	4.3	6.4	7.9
1970						
Total	5.5	3.9	4.9	5.9	7.5	8.3
Primary	4.2	3.4	3.7	4.2	5.3	6.7
1975						
Total	10.4	8.4	9.0	11.1	13.6	15.0
Primary	7.8	7.9	7.1	7.6	9.6	10.0
1980						
Total	16.5	14.5	15.8	16.7	18.0	20.6
Primary	12.1	12.6	11.7	11.8	12.0	16.5
1985						
Total	22.7	16.1	21.2	22.9	26.6	30.7
Primary	16.3	13.8	16.3	15.6	17.2	22.1
1986						
Total	24.1	18.3	21.9	25.3	26.2	32.6
Primary	17.4	16.2	16.9	17.2	17.5	22.5
1987						
Total	24.4	18.5	22.9	23.7	28.3	31.6
Primary	17.4	15.9	16.6	16.8	18.8	22.6

Source: Taffel, 1989, p. 6, National Hospital Discharge Survey data.

between 25 and 29, and women over 35. This indicates that the recent drop in the total cesarean rate was led by changes in treatment of women in these age groups. (As of 1987, however, these downward movements were still offset by increases among other age groups.) Since we have no data after 1987, it is unclear what role variations in treatment by age played in the declining total cesarean rate.

Such large variations in age-specific rates raise the question of whether geographic variations result merely from different maternal age distributions, rather than differences in medical practice. Several studies show they do not. A study by Placek and Taffel (1980) provides age-specific rates for 1970 and 1978 by region. Although the figures themselves are dated, they show that regional differences persist even after controlling for maternal age. Not only did rates for the same age groups vary by region in both years; no two regions had the same pattern, much less the same size of age-specific increases between the two years.

For the most part, regional differences were greater in 1978 than in 1970. The largest gap in 1970 was 8.3 percent for women 40 and above; a low of 5 percent of birthing women aged 40+ in the North Central region (Midwest) had cesareans compared with a high of 13.3 percent in the West. By 1978, however, the difference between the most extreme rates had climbed to 28.2 percent; women over 40 had a rate of 8.0 percent in the South but 36.2 percent in the West. These examples also illustrate the relative variability of birthing experiences among older mothers. Cesarean rates for women over 30 varied tremendously in 1978, while treatment of women under 25 hardly differed at all.

These findings do not prove that differences in the age composition of birthing women across regions do not affect overall rates, but they do show that despite any variations in age composition, medical practice differs as well.

Cesarean delivery rates by age for 13 states and New York City in 1983 are shown in Table 15 (Potrzebowski, 1988). These data reinforce the conclusion that medical treatment varies geographically apart from the effect of maternal age. As would be expected, states show greater variation than do regions. Although rates for younger mothers varied

Table 15

Cesarean Section Delivery Rates in Selected States, by Age of Mother: 1983

	Age of Mother					
State	All	Under 20	20-24	25-29	30-34	35 +
Washington	14.3	10.4	13.3	14.9	16.2	18.1
Minnesota	14.8	11.5	13.5	14.9	16.9	17.9
Wisconsin	15.4	12.3	14.6	15.9	16.8	18.4
Montana	15.5	12.0	13.7	16.7	17.0	21.8
Vermont	17.1	14.8	15.8	16.7	19.6	23.1
Maine	17.9	13.7	17.6	18.3	20.2	21.7
Missouri	19.0	14.4	17.7	20.0	22.2	23.6
Pennsylvania	19.3	14.5	17.8	19.8	22.7	25.0
Connecticut	19.4	14.7	17.5	19.6	21.5	24.8
Georgia	19.6	15.4	18.9	20.8	23.3	26.1
New Hampshire	19.6	15.0	16.8	21.3	21.8	24.6
California	19.8	14.4	17.7	20.4	23.4	26.2
New York City	20.3	12.7	17.4	21.0	23.5	28.8
Maryland	23.2	17.4	21.4	23.8	26.8	29.5

Source: Potrzebowski 1988, III-9

Note: Maryland and Wisconsin data are by state of residence; all others are by state of occurrence.

less than those for older ones, even women under 20 faced quite different probabilities of having a cesarean birth; 10.4 percent in Washington versus 17.4 percent in Maryland. For women 35 and over, the largest gap was between Minnesota with 17.9 percent and Maryland with 29.5 percent.

Age-specific time series are available for four states: Wisconsin between 1968 and 1985 (Kirby, 1987); California between 1960 and 1975 (Petitti et al., 1979); Missouri in 1972 and 1981 (Missouri Division of Health, 1982); and upstate New York for 1968-1969 and 1977-1978 (Zdeb, et al., 1980). These data show the same general patterns as do national data. Older women have higher cesarean rates than younger women, and all age groups have experienced large increases in cesarean rates over time. Also similar is the fact that younger women experienced more rapid increases than older women during the 1960s and 1970s.

In addition, the California and Wisconsin studies present data on the age composition of birthing women. Despite much talk of increasing maternal age, at least at the national level, the proportion of all birthing women in Wisconsin who were in their 30s was lower in 1985 than in 1970. After 1980 there were, however, relatively fewer women giving birth between the ages of 20 and 24, and relatively more between 25 and 29. The proportion under 20 has been falling since 1975. Approximately the same pattern of changes occurred in California. However, the two populations are not quite the same overall age. Given California's high cesarean rate, one might expect its mothers to be slightly older than Wisconsin's. Just the opposite is true; California mothers are a bit younger than Wisconsin mothers. Age composition of these two populations cannot, then, even partially explain the large difference between their overall cesarean rates. In fact, age composition makes the difference even harder to understand based on clinical reasons alone.

PARITY

Another way we might explain geographic variations in cesarean rates is by comparing data on parity. In general, cesarean rates decrease for higher birth orders (Potrzebowski, 1988; Kirby, 1987; Petitti et al., 1979; Williams and Hawes, 1979; Zdeb, et al., 1980). Table 16 presents cesarean rates by parity for 11 states and New York City in 1983 (Potrzebowski, 1988). The rates vary considerably among states and are again highest in Maryland and lowest in Washington, just as they were for rates by maternal age.

Time series data are again available for Wisconsin, California, Missouri, and upstate New York. The most recent data are from Wisconsin (Kirby, 1987). They show that before 1970, rates for all parities (data are for 1st through 5th-plus child) were clustered together around 4 percent to 5 percent. By 1985, rates for each parity had increased substantially and had spread apart; the rate for the first birth was

Table 16

Cesarean Section Delivery Rates in Selected States, by Birth Order: 1983

State	Birth Order					
	All	First	Second	Third	Fourth	Fifth +
Connecticut	19.4	21.5	20.3	18.1	14.3	17.9
Minnesota	14.8	15.6	15.7	13.9	12.4	8.5
Montana	15.5	16.4	16.0	14.2	12.0	12.1
Pennsylvania	19.3	20.6	19.8	17.6	14.5	13.1
Missouri	19.0	20.0	20.0	17.0	14.8	14.8
Washington	14.3	15.2	14.8	13.1	11.4	10.4
Vermont	17.1	16.9	18.1	17.4	13.1	13.1
California	19.8	21.3	20.1	18.6	16.2	14.3
Maryland	23.3	24.3	23.3	21.0	18.9	18.1
New York City	20.3	20.6	21.5	20.0	16.9	15.6
Wisconsin	15.4	16.4	15.4	14.5	13.3	11.4
Georgia	19.6	20.7	20.6	17.8	13.7	13.1

Source: Potrzebowski, 1988, III-14

Note: Maryland and Wisconsin data are by state of residence; all others are by state of occurrence.

highest at about 18.5 percent, and the rate for the fifth-plus birth was lowest--below 14 percent.

Data from upstate New York show some different patterns (Zdeb et al., 1980). While first-parity births also have the highest cesarean rates in 1968-69 and 1977-78, the pattern for subsequent parities is not clear. Data are broken out for whites and nonwhites (nonwhites have higher rates for all except first births), and by parity for both years. In most cases, there is little variation among higher birth orders.

MATERNAL AGE AND PARITY COMBINED

The few studies that analyze the joint effects of maternal age and parity come to the same basic conclusions. Time series of parity and age data are available for California from 1965 to 1975 (Petitti et al., 1979), and for Missouri from 1972 to 1981 (Missouri Division of Health,

1982), allowing us to compare changes in rates by birth order over time. They show that cesarean section rates (1) decreased steadily as parity increased, (2) rose with increasing maternal age, and (3) for every age and parity group, increased over time. Thus, the highest California rate is for women of 40 years and over having their first child in 1975--a full 53 percent. For Missouri, the highest rate is for women 35 and over having their first child in 1981, at 38.8 percent.

For California women under 30, rates for first births increased faster than for second births, which increased faster than for third births. Rates for four-plus births increased the most slowly of all. For women over 35, the pattern was just the opposite; rates for first-parity births increased the most slowly, possibly because they were so high even in 1960, and rates for higher-parity births increased faster. The Missouri data are difficult to interpret in this fashion since parities of three and above are grouped.

Wisconsin rates by parity and age are available for 1984 only and show no surprising patterns. Cesarean rates for each succeeding child dropped in every age group (except under 20, where the sample sizes may have been quite small).

The percentage of total births in California (Petitti et al., 1979) that were of fourth or higher parity decreased sharply from 25.5 percent in 1965 to 12.1 percent in 1975. In Wisconsin this percentage fell from 25.1 percent in 1968 to 10.7 percent in 1977 (Nashold, 1980). Since high-parity births have a lower incidence of cesarean than low-parity births, women's changing reproductive behavior has undoubtedly contributed to increasing cesarean rates in both states.

Questions remain about the effects of diagnosis on these relationships. For example, age, parity, and prior C-section are all correlated. To what extent are age and parity differences in C-section rates due to (or masked by) a higher proportion of prior C-sections among older, higher-parity women? Do the age and parity relationships hold up separately for women with and without prior C-sections? The multivariate studies discussed in the following section help to answer these questions.

5. VARIATIONS RELATED TO OTHER FACTORS AFFECTING CESAREAN RATES

In this section, we summarize the literature on the relation of C-section rates to factors other than the four major diagnoses discussed in Section 3. Diagnoses are *controlled for* in many of the studies reviewed here, but we do not report any further results about the effect of diagnosis on C-section rates, because there are no surprises: Any of the four major diagnoses increases C-section rates. However, we do report additional results concerning the effect of maternal age and parity on C-section rates (discussed in Section 4), because the previous discussion left open questions about the relationships among diagnosis, age, parity, and C-section rates.

Table 17 summarizes the multivariate analyses that we reviewed; Table 18 summarizes bivariate analyses. The multivariate analyses are, we believe, of wider relevance. Multivariate analyses estimate the independent effect of each factor in the equation after controlling for the effects of all of the other factors in the equation. Thus they are less likely to confound the effect of one factor (such as mother's age) with the effects of other factors that may be correlated with it (such as parity, birth weight, or clinical diagnosis).

Both Table 17 and Table 18 are quite sparse, and that is one major finding of this portion of our literature synthesis. With the exception of Tussing and Wojtowycz (1992), there are no studies yet available that estimate simultaneously the effects of a reasonably comprehensive set of clinical, patient, physician, and hospital variables.

Despite substantial differences in the number and choice of variables to include, the multivariate studies summarized in Table 17 provide a consistent picture of the effects of several patient characteristics.

The probability of C-section generally increases with mother's age, and decreases with parity. (Tussing and Wojtowycz also found that very young mothers have higher C-section rates than do those in the most-common childbearing years.) This is true for women without prior C-section (the "primary C-section" columns of the tables) and for women

Table 17

Multivariate Analyses of Nonclinical Factors Affecting Cesarean Rates

	Any c-section		Primary c-section											Secondary c-section		
	S8	D5	Z3	B1	N2	D5	G5	G4	W3	O1	W4	M2	T3	S8	G3	S6
PATIENT																
age			+	+	ns		+	+	+	ns	+	+	-+		ns	+
parity			-	-			-	-	-		-		-			
plurity									+		+		+			
nonwhite			+		+				+			ns	+			+
hispanic							-					ns	+			+
education			-									-	-			
urban or suburban res												+			ns	
income					ns		+						ns			ns
unmarried			+									ns	-			
no prenatal care			+									ns	-			
birth weight							-+		-+		+	-+	-+			
private patient		+				+										
private insurance	+												0	+		0
non-kaiser hmo	+												-	+		
medicaid	0									-			+	+		
kaiser	-													-		
self-pay	-												-	-		-
indigent	-													-		-
PHYSICIAN																
ob/gyn					+								+		ns	
age													ns		+	
sex													ns		ns	
volume															+-	
percent high risk															ns	
c-section rate															+	
referral rate (out)															+	
HOSPITAL																
birth center				-												
size					-				+-	ns	+		ns			-
level of care					+				-			ns	-		-	
proprietary					-						+					0
religious					+											-
kaiser									-		-					-
county									-		-		ns			-
university									-							-
teaching									-	-		ns	-			-
OTHER CONTROL	clin+	clin+		clin	clin	clin+		clin+	breech	clin+	breech	parity	clin+	clin+		clin

ns denotes not significant
\+ denotes a positive or positively sloped relationship
\- denotes a negative or negatively sloped relationship
0 denotes a reference category
-+ denotes an initially negatively then positively sloped relationship (u-shaped)
+- denotes an initially positively then negatively sloped relationship (hill-shaped)
clin indicates that clinical variables were also controlled for
clin+ indicates that clinical and other variables were also controlled for

Table 18

Bivariate Analyses of Nonclinical Factors Affecting Cesarean Rates

	Any c-section					Primary c-section							Secondary c-section		
	Z2	K1	A2	R2	M5	Z3	Z2	A4	E1	H1	N1	M2	Z2	A4	G3
PATIENT															
age	+	+		+			+					+	+		-
parity		-													
plurity															
nonwhite	-	ns		-	-							ns	-		
hispanic												+			
education	+				+							+			
urban or suburban res												+			-
income															
unmarried					-							-			
no prenatal care					-							-			
birth weight		-+										-+			
private patient				+											
from physician family											+				
PHYSICIAN															
ob/gyn															-
age															+
sex															ns
volume															-
percent high risk															+-
c-section rate															+
referral rate (out)															+
"convenience"									+						
HOSPITAL															
birth center															
size	+-					+						ns			
level of care			+-							-		+			-
proprietary	+														
religious															
kaiser															
county	-														
university															
teaching	-					+		+				+		-	

ns denotes not significant
+ denotes a positive or positively sloped relationship
- denotes a negative or negatively sloped relationship
-+ denotes an initially negatively then positively sloped relationship (u-shaped)
+- denotes an initially positively then negatively sloped relationship (hill-shaped)

with prior C-section (the "secondary C-section" columns), and it is true even after controlling for other diagnoses.

The effect of birth weight is also convincingly estimated: Either very low or very high birth weight increases the probability of C-section compared with birth weight in a "normal" range. This result is corroborated by two bivariate studies (Table 18).

Nonwhite race is consistently estimated to increase the probability of C-section in the multivariate studies, and to decrease it in the bivariate studies. Education goes in the other direction; it is negatively related to C-section in the multivariate studies, and positively in the bivariate studies. Race and education are correlated with other variables such as income and type of hospital that may affect probability of C-section, so it is not too surprising that their effects depend on what else is controlled for in the estimated equation.

The evidence on effects of other demographic patient variables, including Hispanic ethnicity, income, marital status, and location of residence, is spotty or mixed.

Three multivariate studies agree that patients enrolled in a Kaiser HMO and self-pay or indigent patients have lower C-section rates than do others. The evidence about the relative C-section rates for patients with other insurance coverages is mixed.

Two multivariate studies suggest that obstetricians tend to do more C-sections than physicians who are not obstetricians. Evidence on the effects of other physician characteristics is weak. Only one study looked at a fairly comprehensive set of physician characteristics; that study (Goldman et al., 1990) did both multivariate and bivariate analyses. However, that study did not control well for clinical or other nonclinical factors, and its results are not supported by Tussing and Wojtowycz (1992) for the three comparable variables.

The multivariate studies agree that Kaiser, county, university, and teaching hospitals all tend to have lower C-section rates. One other multivariate study compares a hospital with a birthing center, and convincingly shows the birthing center to have a lower C-section rate after controlling for clinical factors including diagnosis, patient age, and parity. The estimated effects of size, level of care, and other hospital ownership variables differ among the multivariate studies--depending, presumably, on what hospitals are in the sample and what other correlated factors are controlled for in each study.

6. CONCLUSION

The literature describes dramatic increases in aggregate C-section rates over time, and dramatic differences among countries, regions, states, and smaller areas. The changes over time in the United States can be largely attributed to changes in the four major diagnoses that lead to most C-sections: more-frequent diagnoses of prior C-section, dystocia, and fetal distress; and higher C-section rates for breech diagnoses. But these attributions still fail to explain why C-section rates have increased so dramatically in the last two decades. After all, an increase in prior C-sections is one *result* of the rise in primary C-section rates. Dystocia and fetal distress are diagnosed much more frequently now than in 1970, but that must reflect changing reporting standards more than changing clinical presentations. The literature offers speculations about the reasons for these changes over time, but little or no hard evidence.

Geographic differences are even less well explained than are variations over time. In principle, one could attempt to attribute geographic differences to the four major diagnoses, in the same way that has been done for differences over time. However, no one has yet done such a study, probably because the required data have not been assembled.

A complete understanding of variations in the overall C-section rate would, we believe, require separate predictive models of the probability of each major diagnosis, together with separate models of the probability of C-section, conditional on each of the diagnoses.

We would like to test for the effects on C-section rates of a comprehensive set of clinical, patient, physician, and hospital variables to the extent that data allow. This requires the use of linked data sets. Some important variables, such as parity and birth weight, are available only from the birth certificate. Others, such as detailed clinical diagnoses, are available only on hospital discharge data. Physician and hospital characteristics must be linked in from American Medical Association and American Hospital Association data using physician and hospital codes that are available on the birth certificate or hospital discharge data sets from some but not all states. Tussing and Wojtowycz, 1992, used linked data to study C-section rates in New York State. A better understanding of geographic variations requires that similar studies be done in other states.

APPENDIX A
TOTAL CESAREAN SECTION RATES

Table A.1

Total Cesarean Section Rates, by Year and Geographic Area

Region	Ref	1970	1971	1972	1973	1974	1975	1976	1977	1978	1979	1980	1981	1982	1983	1984	1985	1986	1987	1988	1989	1990
US	N4,P2,P3,T1,T2,V2	5.5	5.8	7.0	8.0	9.2	10.4	12.1	13.7	15.2	16.4	16.5	17.9	18.5	20.3	21.1	22.7	24.1	24.4	24.7	23.8	23.5
	S2	5.7				9.2				14.7						21.2						
	S3										14.1					19.0						
	N3																23					
Midwest	M3,P2,P5,T1	4.7	5.2	5.7	7.0	8.4	9.3	10.6		13.9		14.9			18.8	18.9		23.2	23.2			
	S3															17.1						
IL	G1,G2									14	15	16	17	18	18.7							
IL	S4,V2•																	22.3			21.9	
Chicago, IL	*G1,G2*									*14*	*15*	*16*	*17*	*18*	*18.7*							
IN	S4,V2•																	21			21.2	
IA	S4,V2•																		20.9			18.9
KS	P6	4.3					9.0					16.1			20.7							
KS	S4,V2•																	26.5	27.4		23.7	23.4
KY	V2																				23.6	23.8
MI	G1,G2										9.0	10.0	10.8	11.7	12.7							
MI	S4,V2•																	25			22.9	22.0
Wayne Cty-Detroit, MI	*G1,G2*											*9.9*	*10.8*	*11.4*	*12.3*							
MN	P6	4.3					7.9					13.9			16.3							
MN	S4,V2•																	17.2	19		18.1	17.6
MO	P6	4.7					9.2					15.1			19.0							
MO	M5			6.0									16.1									
MO	G1,G2									13.2	14.1	14.8	15.8	17.3	18.6							
MO	S4,V2•																		24.7	24.5		23.3
St. Louis, MO	*G1,G2*									*12.9*	*13.2*	*13.4*	*13.9*	*16.3*	*16.8*							
NE	G6,G7	5.5	5.7	5.8	7	7.4	8.3	9.6	10.4	11.8	13.1	13.5		15								
NE	V2																					19.6
ND	S4,V2•																		19.8			19.3
OH	S4,V2•																	23.9			25.9	25.7
TX	V2																				25.9	

Table A.1--continued

Region	Ref	1970	1971	1972	1973	1974	1975	1976	1977	1978	1979	1980	1981	1982	1983	1984	1985	1986	1987	1988	1989	1990
WI	N1	5.0	5.4	5.8	6.6	7.5	8.2	9.3	10.4													
WI	K1	5.0	5.4	5.9	6.7	7.6	8.3	9.5	10.6	12.1	12.9	13.6	14.3	15.2	15.8	17.4	17.9					
WI	S4,V2•																	19.2			17.5	17.5
North East	M3,P2,P5,T1	6.2	7.4	7.3	9.0	10.8	11.9	14.6		17.6		19.2			21.5	21.4		25.4	26.4			
	S3															20.2						
CT	P6											18.7			20.7							
CT	S4,V2•																	23.2	24.6			21.9
ME	P6														17.9							
ME	S4,V2•																	22.1	23.1			22.2
MA	M2							13.9	15.3	17.7	19.0	19.0	19.5	20.1								
MA	G1,G2								15.3	17.7	19.0	18.4	19.5	19.4	20.1							
MA	M1																		24.6	24.4		
MA	S4,V2•																	23.7			22.9	
Greater Boston, MA	*G1,G2*								*19.5*	*20.8*	*22.4*	*22.1*	*22.6*	*20.3*	*20.3*							
Winthrop MA	*A1*																*30.4*					
Attleboro MA	*A1*																*28.3*					
Milton MA	*A1*																*30.1*					
Braintree MA	*A1*																*28.0*					
Quincy MA	*A1*																*27.2*					
Lynn MA	*A1*																*26.2*					
Weymouth MA	*A1*																*26.1*					
Springfield MA	*A1*																*24.2*					
Webster MA	*A1*																*17.5*					
Andover MA	*A1*																*18.1*					
Fairhaven MA	*A1*																*16.3*					
Littleboro MA	*A1*																*16.4*					
Millbury MA	*A1*																*14.4*					
North Adams MA	*A1*																*13.5*					
NH	P6									15.0					19.6							
NH	S4,V2•																	23.0	23.3		22.0	22.2†
NJ	H1	6.1	6.8	7.5	8.7	9.9	10.1	13.5	15.1	16.6	18.1	19.5	20.2	21.4	22.0	23.9	24.8	26.7				
NJ	S4,V2•																	26.8			27.0	

Table A.1--continued

Region	Ref	1970	1971	1972	1973	1974	1975	1976	1977	1978	1979	1980	1981	1982	1983	1984	1985	1986	1987	1988	1989	1990
NY	G1,G2								14	16	17	18	19	20.7	20.8							
NY	S4,V2•																24.2	25.8			23.5	23.6
NY City, NY	*34*	*5.0*					*8.3*			*19.1*					*20.4*							
NY City, NY	*G1,G2*									*19*	*20*	*20*	*21*	*22*	*20.3*							
Upstate NY	*34*	*5.7*					*10.3*					*18.9*			*21.8*							
PA	G1,G2								12	9	15	16	17	17.8	18.9							
PA	P6	5.6					10.0					16.0			19.3							
PA	S4,V2•																	22.7	23.9		23.0	21.9
Philadelphia Cty, PA	*G1,G2*								*14*	*9*	*16*	*17*	*18*	*18.8*	*20.6*							
RI	H3																	23.8	23.1	22.4		
RI	V2																				20.8	20.0
VT	P6									13.8		15.0			17.2							
VT	S4,V2•																		20.1		19.1	19.4
South	M3,P2,P5,T1	5.8	5.2	7.4	8.0	9.3	10.5	12.1		15.2		16.8			21.3	22.7		24.8	25.5			
	S3															20.4						
AL	S4,V2•																		17.9		25.7	25.9
AR	S4,V2•																		24.3		27.1	27.8
DE	V2																				26.6	25.3
DC	G1,G2								19	20	22	24	24	27	27.2							
DC	S4,V2•																	30.1	30.3		25.0	26.6
FL	S4,V2•																24.8	27.7	27.9			26.4
GA	G1,G2								13.2	15.6	13.5	15.5	15.9	19.3	19.6							
GA	P6,S4,V2•											15.4			19.9				24.9		23.2	22.3
Atlanta, GA	*G1,G2*								*10.7*	*12.4*	*13.0*	*14.1*	*15.2*	*17.8*	*21.8*							
LA	V2																					27.3
New Orleans, LA	*W2*																*28.2*					
MD*	P6	5.7					12.8					20.6			23.6							
MD	S4,V2•																	26.6	26.4	26.0		24.4
MS	S4,V2•																		26.2			26.3
NC	S4,V2•																			24		23.0
SC	S4,V2•																		23.7			22.8§
TN	S4,V2•																	20.4	20.8		24.4	24.5

Table A.1--continued

Region	Ref	1970	1971	1972	1973	1974	1975	1976	1977	1978	1979	1980	1981	1982	1983	1984	1985	1986	1987	1988	1989	1990
VA	G1,G2										9.3	9.3	13.7	15.0	15.9							
VA	S4,V2•																	19.1	19.2		24.1†	24.1
WV	S4,V2•																		24.6		25.4	26.3
West	M3,P2,P5,T1	5.7	5.7	8.3	8.0	8.1	9.9	11.3		14.6		15.3			19.1	20.6		22.9	22.5			
	S3															18.9						
AZ	S4																		22.2	20.8		
CA	S9	6.9	7.6	8.7	9.9	11.3	12.8	14	15.4	15.7	16.5	17.1	17.3	18.5	20	20.8	21.6	23.1				
CA	W6															20.9	21.7	23.1	23.6	22.9		
CA	V2																				22.9	21.4
CA	W5	6.9	7.6	8.7	9.9	11.3	12.8	14.0	15.4													
CA	G1,G2								15	16	16	17	17	18.4								
CA	P1						12.7															
CA	S7														21.7	22.6	23.2	24.5	25.0			
CA	P6	6.9					12.8					17.1			19.8							
Los Angeles Cty, CA	*G1,G2*								*15*	*16*	*16*	*17*	*17*	*18.3*								
Los Angeles Cty, CA	*34*															*21.0*	*21.7*	*22.9*	*24.5*	*24.1*		
San Diego Cty, CA	*34*															*20.2*	*22.3*	*23.9*	*22.1*	*21.9*		
Orange Cty, CA	*34*															*23.7*	*24.1*	*25.7*	*25.4*	*24.3*		
Santa Clara Cty, CA	*34*															*18.7*	*20.7*	*21.2*	*21.7*	*20.1*		
San Bernardino Cty, CA	*34*															*21.2*	*21.3*	*23.6*	*23.9*	*23.3*		
Alameda Cty, CA	*34*															*20.7*	*21.9*	*22.1*	*22.2*	*21.3*		
Riverside Cty, CA	*34*															*21.6*	*22.0*	*23.2*	*23.6*	*23.2*		
Sacramento Cty, CA	*34*															*18.6*	*18.4*	*20.6*	*20.6*	*20.8*		
Contra Costa Cty, CA	*34*															*25.9*	*25.8*	*26.7*	*26.2*	*24.4*		
San Francisco Cty, CA	*34*															*19.7*	*19.5*	*20.8*	*21.7*	*21.9*		
Ventura Cty, CA	*34*															*22.5*	*23.1*	*24.6*	*24.7*	*23.3*		
Fresno Cty, CA	*34*															*22.0*	*22.5*	*23.8*	*23.5*	*23.9*		
CO	S4																	20.6	20.2			
ID	V2																					18.9
MT	P6	5.0					7.4					12.6			15.5							
MT	S4,V2•																		19.7		20.7	20.9
NV	S4,V2•																		19.2		31.7	
NM	P6											14.7			17.2							
NM	S4,V2•																		20		18.7	18.5

Table A.1--continued

Region	Ref	1970	1971	1972	1973	1974	1975	1976	1977	1978	1979	1980	1981	1982	1983	1984	1985	1986	1987	1988	1989	1990
OR	S4,V2*																		22.4		21.0	
UT	P6									10.1		11.7			13.9							
UT	S4,V2*																	18			18.4	17.9
WA	P6											14.3			16.5							
WA	S4,V2*																		21.9	21.7		21.0
WY	S4,V2*																[18.5	]	[21.2	]	18.5	19.6
HI	S4,V2*																			22.8		20.6
AK	V2																				15.2	15.3
Canada	N4,W1	5.7	6.4	7.2	8.0	9.0	9.6	10.8	12.1	13.9	15.1	15.9	17.0	18.3								
	L2	6.0	6.4	7.2	8.0	9.0	9.6	10.8	12.1	13.9	14.7	15.2	15.8									
	N3															[	19	]				

* Data represent births ocurring to all residents of Maryland regardless of state of delivery.

REFERENCES

A1

Acker, David B.; Haas, Susan; O'Brien, Elizabeth; Donahue, Charles L. Jr.; Porell, Marjorie McGuirk; Sachs, Benjamin P. Cesarean Birth Rate: Small-Geographic-Area Analysis. American Journal of Obstetrics and Gynecology; August 1988; 159(2): 386-388. (Data from the Massachusetts Department of Public Health and the Massachusetts Health Consortium.)

A2

Adams, Jeffrey L. The Use of Obstetrical Procedures in the Care of Low-Risk Women. Women & Health; Spring 1983; 8 (1) p25-34. (Minnesota birth and death certificates of infants born in southeastern Minnesota hospitals.)

A3

Anderson, Geoffrey M; Lomas, Jonathan. Recent trends in cesarean section rates in Ontario [Comment in Can Med Assoc J 1990 Jan 15;142(2):101]. Can Med Assoc J; Nov 15 1989; 141 (10) p1049-53. (Hospital Medical Records Institute data abstracted from hospital discharge records.)

A4

Anderson, Geoffrey M; Lomas, Jonathan. Explaining Variations in Cesarean Section Rates: Patients, Facilities or Policies? Can Med Assoc J; Feb 1 1985; 132 (3) p253-6, 259. (Hospital Medical Records Institute data abstracted from hospital discharge records.)

A5

Anderson, Geoffrey M; Lomas, Jonathan. Determinants of the Increasing Cesarean Birth Rate--Ontario Data 1979 to 1982. New England Journal of Medicine; October 4, 1984; 311(14): 887-892. (Hospital Medical Records Institute data abstracted from hospital discharge records.)

B1

Baruffi, G.; Strobino, DM; Paine, LL. Investigation of institutional differences in primary cesarean birth rates. J Nurse Midwifery; Sep-Oct 1990; 35 (5) p274-81. (Data from a random sample abstracted retrospectively from medical records from a birthing center and a nearby maternity hospital.)

B2

Bergsjo, Per; Schmidt, Eberhard; Pusch, Detlev. Differences in the Reported Frequencies of Some Obstetrical Interventions in Europe. Br J Obstet Gynaecol; Jul 1983; 90 (7) p628-32. (Questionnaire administered by the WHO European Regional Perinatal Study Group to member nations in 1980.)

B3

Bertollini, Roberto; Di Lallo, Domenico; Rapiti, Elisabetta; Perucci, Carlo A. Cesarean Section Rates in Italy [letter to editor re Placek & Taffel, Notzon, Haynes de Regt, etc.]. Am J Publ Hlth; December 1987; 77(12): 1554. (Birth Registration System data.)

B4

Borthen, Ingrid; Lossius, Petter; Skjaerven, Rolv; Bergsjo, Per. Changes in Frequency and Indications for Cesarean Section in Norway, 1967-1984. Acta Obstet Gynecol Scand; 1989; 68 (7) p589-93. (Medical Birth Registry data.)

C1

Chassin et al., "Variations in the Use of Medical and Surgical Services by the Medicare Population," New England Journal of Medicine, January 30, 1986. (No data taken from this source.)

C2

Chattopadhyay, SK; Sengupta, PB; Edrees, YB; Lambourne, A. Cesarean Section: Changing Patterns in Saudi Arabia. Int J Gynaecol Obstet; Oct 1987; 25 (5) p387-94. (Obstetric records from the Maternity and Children's Hospital.)

C3

Collea, Joseph V.; Chein, Connie; Quilligan, Edward J. The Randomized Management of Term Frank Breech Presentation: A Study of 208 Cases. Am J Obstet Gynecol; May 15, 1980; 137(2): 235-244.

D1

Das, B.; Basak, B.; Sengupta, A. Caesarean section (present and past). J Indian Med Assoc; Aug 1984; 82 (8) p276-8. (Records from the Chittaranjan Seva Sadan hospital.)

D2

Davis, Letitia K., et al., Cesarean Births in Massachusetts, Massachusetts Department of Public Health, Division of Health

Statistics and Research, October 1984. (Data from birth certificates.)

D3

DeMott, RK; Sandmire, HF. The Green Bay Cesarean Section Study. I. The Physician Factor as a Determinant of Cesarean Birth Rates. Am J Obstet Gynecol; Jun 1990; 162 (6) p1593-9; discussion 1599-602. (Hospital records of deliveries performed by 11 physicians at two Green Bay hospitals.)

D4

de Muylder, Xavier; Thiery, Michel. The Cesarean Delivery Rate Can Be Safely Reduced in a Developing Country. Obstet Gynecol; Mar 1990; 75 (3 Pt 1) p360-4. (Gweru Hospital records.)

D5

de Regt, Roberta Haynes; Minkoff, Howard L.; Feldman, Joseph; Schwarz, Richard H. Relation of Private or Clinic Care to the Cesarean Birth Rate [also: The Obstetrician's Dilemma--How Much Fetal Monitoring and Cesarean Section Is Enough? (editorial response by Emanuel A. Friedman to de Regt & Leveno articles, same issue)]. New England Journal of Medicine; September 4, 1986; 315(10): 619-624. (Data abstracted from records of four Brooklyn hospitals.)

E1

Evans, Mark I; Richardson, David A; Sholl, John S; Johnson, Barbara A. Cesarean Section--Assessment of the Convenience Factor. J Reprod Med; Sep 1984; 29(9): 670-6. (Data abstracted from records of four Chicago area hospitals.)

G1

Gleicher, Norbert. The Cesarean-Section Epidemic. Mt Sinai J Med (NY); Sep 1986; 53 (7) p563-5. (Data supplied by state government agencies through personal communication.)

G2

Gleicher, Norbert. Cesarean Section Rates in the United States. The Short-Term Failure of the National Consensus Development Conference in 1980 [also see p3295]. JAMA; Dec 21 1984; 252(23): 3273-6. (Data supplied by state government agencies through personal communication.)

G3

Goldman, G.; Pineault, R.; Bilodeau, H.; Blais, R. Effects of patient, physician and hospital characteristics on the likelihood of vaginal birth after previous cesarean section in Quebec. Can Med Assoc J; Nov 15 1990; 143 (10) p1017-24. (Data from MED ECHO, a database containing hospital discharge forms issued in Quebec.)

G4

Gordon, D.; Milberg, J.; Daling, J.; Hickok, D. Advanced maternal age as a risk factor for cesarean delivery. Obstet Gynecol; Apr 1991; 77 (4) p493-7. (Data from certificates of births occurring in King County, Washington.)

G5

Gould, Jeffrey B; Davey, Becky; Stafford, Randall S. Socioeconomic Differences in Rates of Cesarean Section [Comment in N Engl J Med 1990 Jan 25;322(4):268-70]. N Engl J Med; Jul 27 1989; 321 (4) p233-9. (Data from birth certificates of infants born to Los Angeles County residents.)

G6

Grant, RS; Hill, CY. Recent trends in cesarean sections in Nebraska, 1965 to 1978. Nebr Med J; Dec 1981; 66 (12) p270-5. (Data compiled from hospital discharge records of all Nebraska hospitals.)

G7

Grant, RS; Hill, CY; Woods, RE. Trends in cesarean section rates in Nebraska, 1979 through 1982. Nebr Med J; Jan 1985; 70 (1) p12-18. (Data compiled from hospital discharge records of all Nebraska hospitals.)

H1

Halpin, GJ; Rose, E.; Shapiro, E. Trends in cesarean section rates. N J Med; Nov 1989; 86 (11) p867-73. (Data from Maternity Service Reports submitted to Maternal and Child Health Services.)

H2

Haq, CL. Vaginal birth after cesarean delivery. Am Fam Physician; June 1988; 37 (6) p167-71. (No data taken from this source.)

H3

Hollinshead, WH; Buechner, JS. Cesarean section rates in Rhode Island, 1986-1988. R I Med J; Aug 1990; 73 (8) p376-7. (Hospital discharge data reported to the Division of Family Health.)

J1

Jonas, O; Chan, A; MacHarper, T. Caesarean section in South Australia, 1986 [Comment in Aust N Z J Obstet Gynaecol 1990 Feb;30(1):91]. Aust N Z J Obstet Gynaecol; May 1989; 29 (2) p99-106. (Data from the South Australian Perinatal Statistics Collection of 1986.)

K1

Kirby, Russell S. Trends in Cesarean Section Rates Among Wisconsin Resident Births: 1968-1985. Wisc Med J; Oct 1987; 86 (10) p11-15. (Data from the Wisconsin Vital Statistics Registration System.)

K2

Klein, M., (Nov-Dec 1988), "Do Family Physicians 'Prevent' Cesarean Sections? A Canadian Exploration," Family Medicine, 20 (6) p431-6. (Data from the Health Insurance Authorities of each province, and Statistics Canada.)

L1

Linton, Marianne; Borman, Barry; Findlay, John. Caesarean Section: A National Study. New Zealand Med J; Aug 24 1988; 101 (852) p534-5. (National Health Statistics Center public hospital admission/discharge data.)

L2

Lomas, Jonathan, and Murray Enkin, "Variations in Operative Delivery Rates," in Effective Care in Pregnancy and Childbirth, Ian Chalmers, Murray Enkin, and Marc J.N.C. Keirse, eds., Oxford University Press, 1989, p. 1182-1195. (Data from various national agencies plus some previously published data.)

L3

Lopez-Escobar, G; Fortney, JA; Riano-Gamboa, G; Daza, L. Maternity Record: Initial report on a national experience (Colombia). Int J Gynacol Obstet; Jul-1979 Aug 1978; 17 (1) p40-6. (Questionnaire administered to a sample of 40 urban hospitals.)

M1

Massachusetts Department of Public Health. Advance Data--Births 1988. Bureau of Health Statistics, Research & Evaluation; 1989. (Hospital data.)

M2

Massachusetts Department of Public Health. Cesarean Births in Massachusetts [90p]. Boston: Div Health Statistics & Research; Oct 1984. (1981 Massachusetts birth certificate data.)

M3

Metropolitan Life Insurance Company. Costs for cesarean section: regional variations. Statistical Bulletin of the Metropolitan Insurance Company; Jul-Sep 1986; 67 (3) p2-10. (National Hospital Discharge survey data.)

M4

Miller, CF; Sutter, CS. Vaginal birth after cesarean. J Obstet Gynecol Neonatal Nurs; Sep-Oct 1985; 14 (5) p383-9. (No data taken from this source.)

M5

Missouri Division of Health, Department of Social Services, Missouri Monthly Vital Statistics, Vol. 16, No. 6, August 1982. (Missouri 1981 birth certificate data.)

M6

Moldin, Per; Hokegard, Klas-Henry; Nielsen, Thorkild F. Cesarean Section and Maternal Mortality in Sweden 1973-1979. Acta Obstet Gynecol Scand; 1984; 63 (1) p7-11. (Medical birth register of the National Board of Health and Welfare.)

M7

Monheit, Alan G; Resnik, Robert. Cesarean Section: Current Trends and Perspectives. Clin Perinatol; Feb 1981; 8(1): 101-9. (No data taken from this source.)

M8

Mor-Yosef, Shlomo; Samueloff, Arnon; Modan, Baruch; Navot, Daniel; Schenker, Joseph G. Ranking the Risk Factors for Cesarean: Logistic Regression Analysis of a Nationwide Study. Obstet Gynecol; Jun 1990; 75 (6) p944-7. (Hospital records from 30 maternity hospitals.)

M9

Murray-Arthur, F; Correy, JF. A review of primary caesarean sections in Tasmania. Aust N Z J Obstet Gynaecol; Nov 1984; 24 (4) p242-5. (Data from Tasmanian Notification of Birth Forms.)

N1

Nashold, RD. Increase in Cesarean Deliveries in Wisconsin. Wis Med J; Jul 1980; 79 (7) p30-3. (Birth certificate data.)

N2

Newton, Edward R; Higgins, Craig S. Factors Associated with Hospital-Specific Cesarean Birth Rates. J Reprod Med; Jun 1989; 34 (6) p407-11. (Data from the Hospital Cost Utilization Project database obtained from discharge abstracting services. Not nationally representative.)

N3

Notzon, Francis C. International Differences in the Use of Obstetric Interventions. JAMA; Jun 27 1990; 263 (24) p3286-91. (Insurance claims from Statistics, Canada. U.S. National Hospital Discharge Survey and National Natality Study data.)

N4

Notzon, Francis C.; Placek, Paul J.; Taffel, Selma M. Comparisons of National Cesarean-Section Rates [see Bertollini letter, AJPH, Dec 87]. New England Journal of Medicine; February 12, 1987; 316(7): 386-389. (Insurance claims from Statistics, Canada. U.S. National Hospital Discharge Survey and National Natality Study data.)

O1

Oleske DM, Glandon GL, Giacomelli GJ, Hohmann SF. The cesarean birth rate: Influence of hospital teaching status. Health Services Reasearch; August 1991; 26:3:325-337. (1986 Illinois state hospital discharge data.)

P1

Petitti, D.; Olson, RO; Williams, RL. Cesarean section in California--1960 through 1975. Am J Obstet Gynecol; Feb 15 1979; 133 (4) p391-7. (Birth records provided by the Vital Statistics Section of the California Department of Health.)

P2

Placek, Paul J; Taffel, Selma M. Recent patterns in cesarean delivery in the United States. Obstet Gynecol Clin North Am; Dec 1988; 15 (4) p607-27. (National Hospital Discharge Survey data.)

P3

Placek, Paul J; Taffel, Selma M. Vaginal birth after cesarean (VBAC) in the 1980s. Am J Public Health; May 1988; 78 (5) p512-5. (National Hospital Discharge Survey data.)

P4

Placek, Paul J; Taffel, Selma M. The Frequency of Complications in Cesarean and Noncesarean Deliveries, 1970 and 1978. Public Health Rep; Jul-Aug 1983; 98 (4) p396-400. (No data taken from this source.)

P5

Placek, Paul J; Taffel, Selma M. Trends in cesarean section rates for the United States, 1970-78. Public Health Rep; Nov-Dec 1980; 95 (6) p540-8. (National Hospital Discharge Survey data.)

P6

Potrzebowski, Patricia W. Comparison of Cesarean Trends and Pregnancy Outcome in Selected States [36p, figures + tables]. U.S. DHHS/PHS/ CDC. Proceedings of International Collaborative Effort on Perinatal & Infant Mortality [from APHA 1985, Washington, D.C.]. Hyattsville, MD: Natl Ctr Hlth Statistics; Oct 1988: III 3-36. (Data sources unknown.)

R1

Read, Anne W; Waddell, Vivienne P; Prendiville, Walter J; Stanley, Fiona J. Trends in Caesarean Section in Western Australia, 1980-1987. Med J Aust; Sep 17 1990; 153 (6) p318-23. (Data based on computer files of midwives' "Notification of Case Attended" forms completed in Western Australia.)

R2

Renwick, Manoa Y. Caesarean section rates, Australia 1986: Variations at state and small area level. Aust NZ J Obstet Gynaecol; 1991; 31:4:299-304. (1986; numerator from hospital "morbidity" [discharge] data; denominator from birth registration data.)

R3

Rodrigues, Jose. Urban Hospital Cesarean Section Delivery Rates in Paraiba State, Brazil, 1977-81. Am J Public Health; Jun 1988; 78 (6) p704-5. (Hospital discharge data from the Instituto Nacional de Assistencia Medica da Previdencia Social.)

S1

Sheehan, K Harnett. Caesarean Section for Dystocia: A Comparison of Practices in Two Countries [& April 87 letters]. Lancet; Mar 7 1987; 1 (8532) p548-51. (No data taken from this source.)

S2

Shiono, Patricia H; McNellis, Donald; Rhoads, George G. Reasons for the Rising Cesarean Delivery Rates: 1978-1984. Obstet Gynecol; May 1987; 69 (5) p696-700. (Commission of Professional and Hospital Activities data on member hospitals.)

S3

Shiono, Patricia H.; Fielden, Judy G.; McNellis, Donald; Rhoads, George G.; Pearse, Warren H. Recent Trends in Cesarean Birth and Trial of Labor Rates in the United States. Journal of the American Medical Association; January 23-30, 1987; 257(4): 494-497. (Data from own survey based on a national probability sample stratified by the number of births per hospital.)

S4

Silver, Lynn, and Sidney M. Wolfe, Unnecessary Cesarean Sections: How to Cure a National Epidemic, Public Citizen Health Research Group, Washington D.C., 1989. (State agencies computed and reported these data based on either hospital discharges or birth certificates.)

S5

Singh, Jatiswar; Singh, Manglem; Devi, Bidhumukhi; Devi, Lakshmi; Singh, Indrakumar. A Study of 812 Caesarean Sections with Special Reference to Social Customs and Cultural Traditions of Manipur. J Obstet Gyn India; 1981; 31: 603-7. (Data from a prospective study using hospital records and own survey questionnaire.)

S6

Stafford, Randall S. The Impact of Nonclinical Factors on Repeat Cesarean Section. JAMA; Jan 2 1991; 265 (1) p59-63. (Hospital discharge data collected by the Office of Statewide Health Planning and Development in California.)

S7

Stafford, Randall S. Recent trends in cesarean section use in California. West J Med; Nov 1990; 153 (5) p511-14. (Hospital discharge data collected by the Office of Statewide Health Planning and Development in California.)

S8

Stafford, Randall S. Cesarean Section Use and Source of Payment: An Analysis of California Hospital Discharge Abstracts. Am J Public Health; Mar 1990; 80 (3) p313-15. (Hospital discharge data collected by the Office of Statewide Health Planning and Development in California.)

S9

Stafford, Randall Scott, Source of Hospital Payment as a Determinant of Cesarean Section Use, California, 1986, MS Thesis in Health and Medical Sciences, UC Berkeley, 1988. (Hospital discharge data collected by the Office of Statewide Health Planning and Development in California.)

S10

Stewart, Paula J.; Dulberg, Corinne; Arnill, Ann Chapman; Elmslie, Thomas; Hall, Philip F. Diagnosis of Dystocia and Management with Cesarean Section Among Primiparous Women in Ottawa-Carleton [comment in Can Med Assoc J, 1990 Jun 1 142(11) 1187-8]. Canadian Medical Association Journal; March 1, 1990; 142(5): 459-463. (Discharge data from five hospitals.)

T1

Taffel, Selma M. Cesarean Section in America: Dramatic Trends, 1970 to 1987. Stat Bull Metrop Insur Co; Oct-Dec 1989; 70 (4) p2-11. (National Hospital Discharge Survey data.)

T2

Taffel, Selma M; Placek, Paul J; Liss, T. Trends in the United States cesarean section rate and reasons for the 1980-85 rise. Am J Public Health; Aug 1987; 77 (8) p955-9. (National Hospital Discharge Survey data.)

T3

Tussing AD, Wojtowycz MA. The cesarean decision in New York State, 1986: Economic and noneconomic aspects. Medical Care; June 1992; 30(6):529-540. (1986 birth certificate and supplemental data for upstate New York.)

V1

VandenBroek, N; VanLerberghe, W; Pangu, K. Cesarean sections for maternal indications in Kasongo (Zaire). Int J Gynaecol Obstet; Apr 1989; 28 (4) p337-42. (Kasongo Hospital records.)

V2

VanTuinen, Ingrid, and Sidney M. Wolfe, Unnecessary Cesarean Sections: Halting a National Epidemic, Public Citizen's Health Research Group, 1992. (Survey of health agencies in 48 states. Data based either on hospital discharges or birth certificates. National data are from the National Center for Health Statistics.)

W1

Wadhera, S.; Nair, C. Trends in cesarean section deliveries, Canada, 1968-1977. Can J Public Health; Jan-Feb 1982; 73 (1) p47-51. (Data source unknown.)

W2

Wightkin, Joan H; Lambert, Linda M. Cesarean Childbirth Rate Among Women in the New Orleans Area. J LA State Med Soc; Jul 1988; 140 (7) p39-45. (Own survey of New Orleans hospitals.)

W3

Williams, Ronald L; Chen, Peter M. Controlling the Rise in Cesarean Section Rates by the Dissemination of Information from Vital Records. Am J Public Health; Aug 1983; 73(8): 863-7. (Birth and death certificates for California.)

W4

Williams, Ronald L, Chen, Peter M. Standardized cesarean section rates in California: 1978-1980. Community and Organization Research Institute, UC, Santa Barbara. October 1982 draft. (1978-80 California matched birth and death vital statistics data.)

W5

Williams, Ronald L; Hawes, WE. Cesarean section, fetal monitoring, and perinatal mortality in California. Am J Public Health; Sep 1979; 69 (9) p864-70. (Data from own survey plus linked birth and death records.)

W6

Williams, Ronald, and Roger Wroblewski, 1984-1988: Maternal and Child Health Data Base, Community and Organization Research Institute, UC Santa Barbara, December 1991. (Maternal and Child Health Data Base.)

Z1

Zahniser SC, Kendrick LS, Franks AL, Saftlas AF. Trends in obstetric operative procedures, 1980 to 1987. AJPH; October 1992; 82:10:1340-1344. (National Hospital Discharge Survey.)

Z2

Zdeb, Michael S; Logrillo, Vito M. Cesarean Childbirth in New York State: Trends and Directions. Birth; Dec 1989; 16 (4) p203-7; discussion 207-8. (Upstate New York birth certificate data.)

Z3

Zdeb, Michael S; Therriault, GD; Logrillo, Vito M. Cesarean sections in upstate New York, 1968-1978. Am J Epidemiol; Sep 1980; 112 (3) p395-403. (Upstate New York birth certificate data.)

RECENT STUDIES NOT REVIEWED

Braveman PE, Edmonston S, and Verdon M. Racial/ethnic differences in the likelihood of cesarean delivery, California Am J Pub Health. 1995; 85: 625-630.

Burns LR, Geller SE, and Wholey DR. The effect of physician factors on the cesarean section decision. Medical Care; April 1995; 33 (4) p365-382.

Francome C and Savage W. Cesarean section in Britain and the United States: 12% or 24% is either the right rate? Soc Sci Med (37) 1993; 1199-1218.

Goldman G, Pineault R, Potvin L, et al. Factors influencing the practice of vaginal birth after cesarean section. American Journal of Public Health; August 1993; 83 (8) p1104-1108.

Haas JS, Udvarhelyi S, Epstein AM. The effect of health coverage for uninsured pregnant women on maternal health and the use of cesarean section. JAMA. 1993; 270 (1): 61-64.

McKenzie L, and Stephenson PA. Variation in cesarean section rates among hospitals in Washington State. American Journal of Public Health; August 1993; 83 (8) p1109-1112.

Parrish KM, Holt VL, Easterling TR, et al. Effect of changes in maternal age, parity, and birth weight distribution on primary cesarean delivery rates. JAMA; February 9, 1994; 271 (6) p443-447.

Read AW, Prendiville WJ, Dawes VP, and Stanley FJ. Cesarean section and operative vaginal delivery in low-risk primiparous women, Western Australia. American Journal of Public Health. 1994; 84 (1) 37-42.

Rock SM. Variability and consistency of rates of primary and repeat cesarean sections among hospitals in two states. Public Health Reports. 1993; 108 (4): 514-516.

Sanchez-Ramos L, Moorhead RI, and Kaunitz AM. Cesarean section rates in teaching hospitals: A national survey. Birth. 1994; 21:4.

Tussing, AD and Wojtowycz MA. The effect of physician characteristics on clinical behavior: Cesarean section in New York State. Social Science & Medicine; 1993; 37 (10) p1251-1260.